Critical Praise for Previous Editions

"*. . . a very highly recommended addition to any family, health clinic, medical center, or community library parenting and health/medicine reference collection.*"
–– Jim Cox, Editor, **Midwest Book Review**

"*. . . the most complete collection of vaccine resources for the consumer.*"
— Kristine Severyn, R.Ph., Ph.D., Director, The Vaccine Policy Institute as reviewed in **CCL Family Foundations**

"*. . . doctors can share it with their patients in explaining their views and helping them make informed healthcare decisions.*"
— **Today's Chiropractic**

"*It's great. . . I highly recommend it.*"
— Dr. Tedd Koren, D.C., **The Chiropractic Journal**

"*Your guide is 'perfect'.*"
— Dr. Lawrence Stern, D.C., New York

"*If you have any doubts on this issue get this book and become informed.*"
— Jan Warner-Pooler, Editor, **MAH!**

"*[Ms. Rozario's] time and effort will make your research easier and more productive.*"
–– Barbara Klapperich Senn, Editor, **Family Friends**

"*Diane Rozario has done an excellent job putting this resource guide together, which can be an asset to all those interested in continuing their research on this controversial subject.*"
— Kathy Arnos, **Whole Life Times**

Critical Praise for Previous Editions

"Your Resource Guide has been an INVALUABLE guide for my family. I have told numerous people to purchase it as they search to make an informed decision on vaccinations."
— Judy Vartelas, parent, NJ

"An impressive cross-section of organizations and books dedicated to informing people about the advantages and disadvantages of childhood immunizations. The book reviews are clear, concise, and make it much easier to order."
— Jamie Murphy, author of WHAT EVERY PARENT SHOULD KNOW ABOUT CHILDHOOD IMMUNIZATION

". . . a handy reference guide to information available on all aspects of childhood immunizations."
— Dr. William Campbell Douglass, M.D., Editor, **Second Opinion**

"The [book] also offers information on ordering books that are still in print from national and international vaccination and health organizations; important addresses and phone numbers; how to report vaccine injury; and reviews of periodicals."
— Corinne O. Nelson, **Library Journal**

"Thanks for sorting through all this information for all of us."
— Sandra Jamrog, MA, CCE, Childbirth Educator, NY

"It catalogs a full range of opinions and facts – both pro and con – on this controversial issue."
— Jill Cohen, midwife, **Midwifery Today**

". . . the book provides detailed reviews of other publications that address health issues involved in modern vaccinations."
— **Today's Librarian**

THE IMMUNIZATION RESOURCE GUIDE

THE IMMUNIZATION RESOURCE GUIDE

Where to Find Answers to All Your Questions About Childhood Vaccinations

Fourth Edition

By
Diane Rozario

Patter Publications   Burlington, Iowa

Published by
Patter Publications
P.O. Box 204, Burlington, IA 52601
319-752-0039   888-513-7770 (toll free)   208-361-8889 fax
email: patterpublications@yahoo.com
http://www.patterpublications.com

Printed in the United States of America by Morris Publishing,
3212 E. Hwy 30, Kearney, NE 68847, 800-650-7888

Rozario, Diane, 1963 –
    The immunization resource guide: where to find answers to all your
questions about childhood vaccinations/Diane Rozario.
— Fourth edition.
    p.   cm.
    Index.
    ISBN 0-9643366-5-0
    1. Immunization of children—Popular works. 2. Communicable
diseases in children. 3. Infant care.   I. Rozario, Diane.   II Title.
2000
614.4'7—dc20   00-091401

Library of Congress Control Number: 00-091401

ISBN 0-9643366-5-0

DISCLAIMER:

The author is not a medical or legal professional. The information
contained in this Guide is not meant to represent or replace medical or
legal advice. If medical or legal advice is required, the services of a
competent professional should be sought.

Contents

Introduction

The Truth About Vaccines

Vaccines. Medicine's greatest miracle or our immune system's greatest menace?

I imagine that you are reading this book because you have heard some things about vaccinations that have left you wondering. Perhaps a friend has told you that her child screamed for hours after receiving a DTP shot. Or maybe you listened to one of the recent news stories featuring parents upset over the huge number of shots their children must receive. Maybe you know about the congressional hearings held in April 2000 that allege a connection between the MMR vaccine and the onset of autism. Or maybe you heard that the new rotavirus vaccine was recalled in the Fall of 1999 when some children were left with life threatening bowel obstructions after receiving the vaccine. You're wondering if other vaccines may cause health problems too, if not immediately, then down the road.

However, your doctor reassures you that yes, while it is true vaccines can cause problems in some children, this is very rare and your children are in much greater danger if you delay or forego vaccines.

Who are you to believe? What is the truth about vaccines?

Well, you are not alone in your wonderings. In the course of the eight years since I have written the first edition of this guide, there has been a large increase in the number of parent-initiated vaccine organizations around the U.S. These groups all have in common a strong desire to do what's best for their children's health. They want to know more about vaccines than either the two main "sides" in this issue have presented in the past: vaccines are either "magic bullets" or "poison darts". They want scientifically valid information that they can use to make their own informed choice, whatever that choice may ultimately be, either to receive all vaccines, some vaccines, or no vaccines. They want their decision to be a truly knowledgeable one.

This book will help you, if you too seek to make an informed choice about vaccinations.

I am a parent, and like you, I have been faced with making a decision regarding vaccinations for my own children. It hasn't been an easy one, partly because the information that I needed to make an informed decision was sometimes difficult to locate. With the advent of the internet age, it is easier to find information. In fact, the opposite situation is now a problem: having too much information! This Guide battles the "information overload" by categorizing the major aspects of the vaccine issue.

The over 90 book reviews contained in this Guide are divided by topic. The authors range from staunchly pro-vaccine to staunchly anti-vaccine to all views in between. The resource section contains over 130 organizations and publishers. While they may differ in their beliefs, all of the authors and organizations share a sincere interest in the health and welfare of children.

I have added reviews of over a dozen new books to this edition. There are a large number of new vaccine organizations listed. Many of the organizations I list now have websites, making it fast and easy for you to do your own research.

I think you will find this Guide immensely helpful, whether you are just beginning your research, or have already made substantial progress. It is also valuable as a reference for health professionals who wish to better address their patients' questions.

I find vaccines an utterly fascinating topic because of its combination of medicine and government, money and politics. I hope that this book gives you a firm foundation as you start your journey toward understanding this issue and that in the end we all find out the "truth about vaccines". May God bless you and your family with good health.

Diane Rozario

The Vaccination Decision

T he following pages are not meant to be a full treatment of vaccination. However, I felt that some basic information would be helpful in making your decision.

The Childhood Vaccines in Use Today

I explain how the universally recommended childhood vaccines are manufactured. I find that this information is lacking or inaccurate in many vaccination books I have read. (I gratefully acknowledge the use of Drs. Paul Offit's and Louis Bell's book *What Every Parent Should Know About Childhood Vaccines*, reviewed in Section A.1, for help in preparing this information.)

Inactivated Bacterial Vaccines

DTP

Diphtheria, pertussis, and tetanus are all caused by bacteria. Pertussis is caused by the bacterium *Bordetella pertussis*. The bacterium releases a protein, called a toxin, which causes pertussis. Proteins inside the bacterium also cause the disease. The whole-cell, killed pertussis vaccine contains the toxins and the whole bacterium that have been killed by using formaldehyde. The new acellular pertussis vaccine does not contain the whole bacterium. Instead, the toxins that are inside the bacterium are removed and purified. These are then combined with the toxins released by the bacteria to make the acellular pertussis vaccine (aP).

   Diphtheria is caused by a toxin released by the bacterium *Corynebacterium diphtheriae*. The diphtheria vaccine contains the purified toxin, which has formaldehyde added to it to inactivate it (that is, kill it). An inactivated toxin is called a toxoid. Diphtheria vaccine is really a toxoid.

Tetanus is also caused by a toxin released by a bacterium. The bacterium is called *Clostridium tetani*. As with the diphtheria vaccine, the tetanus vaccine is made from the toxin that has been purified and had formaldehyde added to inactivate it. It is called tetanus toxoid. Toxoids are one type of vaccine.

The vaccines in DPT are "inactivated" meaning that the bacteria do not grow in the body once the person is vaccinated. These are the "conventional" methods of bacterial vaccine manufacturing.

The current recommended schedule for the diphtheria, pertussis, and tetanus vaccines combined together as DPT vaccine (also called DTP) is a primary series at two, four, and six months of age with boosters between 12 to 18 months and between 4 to 6 years of age. DPT is not administered from age 7 on, because of the high rate of adverse reactions to the pertussis component. Only TD or Td is used after this age. In general, inactivated vaccines are administered intramuscularly. The combined vaccine using acellular pertussis vaccine is referred to as DTaP. The acellular pertussis vaccine has been approved for use in the U.S. in all five doses of DTaP as of July 1996. Prior to this, DTaP was only allowed for use in the 4th and 5th doses, having been approved for this use in December 1991.

Live Viral Vaccines

Polio

Polio, measles, mumps, and rubella are all caused by viruses. Oral polio vaccine (Sabin vaccine or OPV) is a live virus vaccine composed of three different strains of polio. It is given through the mouth in the same manner as one would encounter the virus naturally. The injected, killed-virus polio vaccine (IPV) has been infrequently used since the 1950's because it was not as effective as OPV. That has recently changed. Because the only cases of paralytic polio now occurring in the U.S. are from people coming in contact with the stool of someone recently vaccinated with the oral polio vaccine, the CDC and AAP have changed their recommendations for this vaccine. As of 1997, the CDC recommended the use of IPV for the first two doses of vaccine at two and four months of age followed by two doses of OPV one to be given between 6 and 18 months of age and the other between 4 to 6 years of age. Effective January 2000, the CDC changed its recommendations again. It now recommends that IPV be given for all four doses.

The poliovirus spreads from the intestines to the nervous system, where it can cause paralysis. Viruses can only grow in live cells. They can not be cultured in medium like bacteria. The oral polio vaccine is grown in cell cultures. After the virus has been grown for a long time in cell cultures it gets better at growing there than in the nervous system because the virus has genetically mutated to adapt to growing in these cells. It is only when poliovirus leave the intestines and enters the nervous system that paralysis can result. OPV creates antibodies mainly in the intestines.

IPV is made differently. The virus is inactivated (that is, killed) by using formaldehyde. Since IPV is given as a shot it increases the number of antibodies in the bloodstream, but creates less in the intestines. Wild-type poliovirus only enters the bloodstream after infecting the intestines. Therefore antibodies from the IPV vaccine can't kill the virus until it has spread from the intestines to the bloodstream.

MMR

Vaccines for measles, mumps, and rubella are combined together into one vaccine called MMR. These are also live viral vaccines. Measles and mumps virus is grown in cells from chick embryos. Rubella virus is grown in human fibroblast cells. Fibroblasts are cells that hold body tissues together. After the virus grows in the cells many times (called "passaging") the virus adapts and becomes better at growing in these cells than in the human cells they usually infect. The virus in the vaccine is still alive but it is weak now and can only grow poorly. This weakening is called attenuation. The MMR vaccine and, generally all live viral vaccines, is injected subcutaneously (i.e., just below the skin). The current recommended schedule for MMR vaccine is a first dose between 12 to 15 months of age with a booster between 4 to 6 years or 11 to 12 years of age.

Chickenpox

Chickenpox is caused by the varicella virus. The chickenpox vaccine (also called varicella zoster vaccine) has been cultured, or "passaged through" human embryonic lung tissue, embryonic guinea pig fibroblasts, and human diploid cells (WI-38 cells taken from an aborted fetus). Diploid cells are normal cells with 46 chromosomes. As with the MMR vaccine, as the varicella virus gets better at growing in these cells it can not grow as well in the human cells it usually infects. The current recommended schedule for chickenpox vaccine is one dose any time after 12 months of age, usually between 12 to 18 months of age, or at 11 to 12 years of age if no dose has been received previously and the child does not have a history of chickenpox.

Because the viruses in these vaccines are attenuated (weakened) before being made into vaccines they should not cause the disease after administration. In order to produce an immune response, live viral vaccines must grow in your body. The weakened virus takes time to grow which is why adverse reactions from an MMR vaccine may not occur until 5 to 12 days after vaccination.

These are the "conventional" methods for live viral vaccine manufacturing.

New Generation Vaccines

I make the distinction between "conventional" vaccines and "new generation" vaccines to highlight the difference in the technology used in their manufacture. The new generation vaccines utilize the many breakthroughs in molecular biology and genetic engineering.

Hib

The first "new generation" vaccine in widespread use is the Hib vaccine. *Haemophilus influenzae* type B (Hib) is a common cause of bacterial meningitis in infants. The Hib vaccines in use now are polysaccharide conjugate vaccines. The Hib bacterium is coated with a sugar called polysaccharide. The body needs to produce antibodies to this sugar to become immune to Hib bacteria. Unfortunately, children under age two can not produce antibodies to this sugar, which is why they can catch this disease more than once as infants. The Hib vaccines available in the early 1980's were not effective for children younger than two, for this reason. The current Hib vaccines, available since 1990, join the sugar to a protein carrier. Doing this allows children under two to be able to make antibodies to the sugar. This joining is called "conjugating". Protein

carriers in use are tetanus toxoid, diphtheria toxoid, and meningcoc-
cal protein. (In an earlier edition of this book I incorrectly stated that
the whole bacteria was joined to the protein carrier and contained in
the vaccine. I apologize for this error. Only the sugar molecules on
the outside of the bacteria are included in the vaccine.)

The current recommended schedule for Hib vaccine is a primary
series at 2, 4, and 6 months of age with a booster between 12 to 15
months of age.

Pneumococcus

Streptococcus pneumoniae, a bacterium, is a leading cause of
bacterial meningitis and acute ear infections in children under the
age of two. There are 90 identified types of this bacterium, called
serotypes; however, a relatively few number of these serotypes are
responsible for the majority of serious infections. Previously a
S.pneumoniae vaccine was available using 23 of these serotypes,
called 23-valent pneumococcal polysaccharide vaccine (PPV23 or
PNU-IMUNE 23). This vaccine, like the earlier Hib vaccine, was
not conjugated and was only effective in children over the age of 2
years. Similar to Hib, *S.pneumoniae* is coated with a sugar, preventing children under two from producing antibodies to it. A new 7-
valent pneumococcal conjugate vaccine (PREVNAR) was licensed
by the FDA in February 2000. As with Hib vaccine, the sugar has
been joined to a protein carrier (diphtheria toxoid) allowing children
under two to make antibodies to it. It is recommended by the CDC
for all children ages 2, 4 , and 6 months, and age 2 years.

Hepatitis B

The other new generation vaccine now in widespread use is a viral
vaccine: hepatitis B. Hepatitis B virus is coated with a surface protein (antigen). This antigen is what makes one sick. The first version
of hepatitis B vaccine was made from the purified surface protein
taken from the blood of people infected with hepatitis B. This
vaccine was called "Heptavax-B" and manufactured by Merck from
1981-1991. It was never approved for use on a mass scale and was
discontinued because of concerns about using a vaccine containing
human blood products.

The new vaccines are genetically engineered recombinant DNA
vaccines. DNA from *E. coli* bacteria are used to transfer the gene

portion of the hepatitis B virus that codes for the surface protein (antigen), into the genetic code of yeast cells. The gene for the antigen is then "expressed" (i.e., grows) in the yeast. The antigen is separated from the yeast and purified. This is made into the vaccine. The current recommended schedule for hepatitis B is a dose at birth, a second dose between 1 to 4 months of age, and a third dose between 6 to 18 months of age or three doses at 11 to 12 years of age, if none have been received previously. In July 1999, the CDC suspended the recommendation to give the hepatitis B vaccine to newborns, when research showed that the combined amounts of thimerosal (a mercury derivative used in childhood vaccines as a preservative) contained in vaccines received by infants before the age of six months exceeded EPA guidelines. A thimerosal-free hepatitis B vaccine was made available in Fall 1999, and the CDC reinstated their recommendation to vaccinate newborns with this vaccine. (Please note that other vaccines still contain thimerosal, see Pediatric Vaccines in Resources (7) for more information.)

Rotavirus

Rotavirus infects the intestines and causes terrible diarrhea. A vaccine for rotavirus was recommended for use in all children in August 1998. Different rotavirus strains infect different animals. However, a strain that is good at infecting one mammal is poor at infecting a different mammal. To make the rotavirus vaccine, "RotaShield", rhesus monkey rotavirus was combined with human rotavirus. This is called a combination or reassortant virus. Doing this makes the human part of the virus weaker so it is not able to infect our body very well, but it can still stimulate the body to produce antibodies.

The CDC suspended the use of the rotavirus vaccine on July 16, 1999 after over 20 children contracted a life threatening bowel obstruction after being vaccinated. The CDC became aware of this problem from VAERS reports. After the CDC announcement many more reports were made to VAERS as doctors and parents looked at medical records and found a connection. As of this writing, around 100 cases of bowel obstruction were under investigation as being caused by the vaccine. The manufacturer, Wyeth-Ayerst Labs, recalled the vaccine in October 1999.

Who is High-Risk for Adverse Reactions?

Parents should be aware of existing health conditions that may make certain vaccines unsuitable for their children. These conditions are called contraindications. Contraindications include allergies to a vaccine component, a neurological condition, a personal history of seizures, an impaired immune system, and a previous severe reaction to a particular vaccine.

However, the rules on what are considered acceptable medical contraindications are constantly changing. They are getting narrower and narrower and excluding more and more conditions. If your child is currently in a high-risk category, you may suddenly find that your child's health condition is no longer considered a valid medical reason to refuse a vaccine. For example, it had always been considered that any child with a severe allergy to eggs should not receive the MMR vaccine, because the vaccine is cultured in chick embryos. However, now it is recommended that these children be immunized with caution, apparently so they will not be denied the benefits of vaccination.

What is a parent to do? You must decide whether or not to take the risk of vaccinating. Use your own best judgment and discuss your situation with your doctor. Pray. Some of the books reviewed in this Guide provide detailed information about contraindications (in particular, see Section A and Section B) and can help you in your decision-making.

Short-Term Adverse Reactions

There are many adverse reactions associated with vaccines. The whole-cell killed pertussis vaccine (the "P" in DTP) has had many short-term adverse reactions reported. Common reactions include fever, fretfulness, pain and swelling at the injection site, and excessive tiredness. Other more severe reactions include high-pitched screaming, convulsions, shock, neurological damage, and even death. These latter are considered rare, though that depends upon which studies you read. Actual reaction rates are unknown, as the reporting system is voluntary and many reactions are never reported.

Long-Term Adverse Reactions

This area is speculative; however, evidence is mounting to support theories of long-term adverse consequences to vaccines. For example, Harris Coulter documents in his book, *Vaccination, Social Violence and Criminality* (reviewed in Section B.2) the supposed link between the whole-cell, killed pertussis vaccine and the current crop of learning disorders, ADD, autism, and other neurological problems prevalent in children today.

Parents and some doctors cite reactions to the hepatitis B vaccine and the MMR vaccine as a factor in the steep rise in autism cases during the 1990's, as well as other neurological and autoimmune diseases, including diabetes (See Section B.4).

The National Childhood Vaccine Injury Act of 1986

Like all medical procedures, vaccines are not without their risks. Who is liable if something happens to your child? Some public health clinics require you to sign a waiver absolving them of all liability if something goes wrong.

In an effort to reduce the number of lawsuits filed against vaccine manufacturers, Congress passed the National Childhood Vaccine Injury Act in 1986 (NCVIA). This law created the National Vaccine Injury Compensation Program (NVICP) so parents can file a claim for compensation through the government (see Section G.1 for details on this program). Parents must first waive their right to sue the vaccine manufacturer before they can file a claim. The program is funded by heavy excise taxes on vaccines.

Your Doctor's Responsibility

With the passage of the NCVIA, your doctor is now required by law to adhere to the following vaccine safety procedures:

You must be given Vaccine Information Statements (VISs) which discuss the diseases and vaccines prior to your child's vaccination and have any and all questions answered. (See Section A.2

for a complete description of the VISs.) The vaccine manufacturer's name and the lot number of the vaccine, as well as the date administered, where it was administered, and by whom must be recorded in the patient's permanent medical record.

Certain serious adverse events, which occur after particular vaccines and within specified time periods, must be reported to health authorities by law. Your doctor should have a copy of the current Vaccine Injury Table, which lists the reactions that must be reported. If your doctor does not have this information, you can request a copy of the current Vaccine Injury Table from the Division of Vaccine Injury Compensation (see "Vaccine Injuries" in Resources). Other adverse events need only be reported voluntarily. You can file a report yourself. (See the Vaccine Adverse Event Reporting System (VAERS) in "Vaccine Injuries" in Resources.)

It is for informed parents to see to it that these safety procedures are followed. The purpose of these procedures is to monitor the safety of vaccines and in particular, to locate "hot lots" of a vaccine which may be causing large numbers of serious reactions. The National Vaccine Information Center (NVIC) keeps track of "hot lots" of certain vaccines and can provide you with these lot numbers so you can avoid giving these to your child (see "Vaccination Organizations" in Resources).

Mandatory Vaccinations

Vaccinations are mandatory for public school admittance in all fifty states. The required vaccines vary from state to state. Hib, hepatitis B, and now, chickenpox are being added to the list of compulsory immunizations in many states.

There are several ways to obtain copies of your state immunization laws. Check your local library for the State Code (it contains all state laws and regulations) and find the section pertaining to immunization. Laws change frequently. Make sure that you have the current ones. Your local health department can also provide you with the list of required vaccinations.

Why are Vaccinations Mandatory?

Vaccination is viewed by the medical community as a public health action that costs little dollar-wise and protects millions from the ravages of epidemic infectious diseases. Beyond money concerns, vaccinations are promoted as a social duty to our nation's children to protect them against disease by forcing their ignorant or negligent parents who, if they were better informed or cared more, would voluntarily accept vaccination. Therefore, according to this argument, vaccination is in our children's best interests and thus should be mandated by law.

Of course, it is true that the state has the right to act for the good of all its citizens. Nobody wants to go to war and die, but someone must be willing to protect our country. In order to protect the majority, a few may suffer from severe adverse effects of vaccinations. The sacrifices made by these few individuals are the price we pay to protect the health of the many. Of course, no parent wants his or her child to be the one to pay the price.

Is this argument still valid? Was it ever valid? In a war everyone knows there is a good chance of death or serious injury. Is this true when we subject ourselves or our children to vaccinations? Are we told all the possible risks beforehand? Are epidemics a threat to us today in our country? Why, if only 50% of children under age two were vaccinated in 1993, as the Clinton Administration asserted at the time, albeit, incorrectly, did we not see infectious disease epidemics ravaging the other 50%?

Legal Exemptions from Receiving Vaccinations

Legal exemptions from vaccinations are allowed in every state. There are three categories: medical, religious, and philosophical. All states allow medical exemptions. All states except West Virginia and Mississippi allow religious exemptions. Around 17 states allow philosophical exemptions. If you are interested in obtaining a legal exemption, it is crucial that you read and thoroughly understand your state's laws (see Section F and "Legal Exemptions" in Resources).

Medical Exemption

For a medical exemption, a medical doctor must sign a waiver. Some states allow osteopaths to sign the waiver. Many states do not allow chiropractors, naturopaths, or other "non-conventional" doctors to sign exemptions because many of these doctors oppose vaccinations. You must check the wording of your state law. A medical waiver can be for only one vaccine (e.g., pertussis), for several vaccines, or for all vaccines. It may be a temporary or permanent exemption. A medical exemption is usually given because a child has had a severe reaction to a previous shot (usually DPT) or is in a high-risk category for possible severe reactions. Unfortunately, many doctors are reluctant to sign these waivers.

Religious Exemption

Some states require that in order to qualify for a religious exemption, you must be a practicing member of an established religion that opposes immunization. This is being challenged in court because it is unconstitutional (see Section F). Other states allow personal religious beliefs to qualify. Again, check the wording of your state law. Generally, to use this exemption you must oppose all vaccinations, not just some. Most states require that you submit a notarized affidavit or a special form signed and notarized to qualify for this exemption.

Philosophical Exemption

This is always changing. At this time, 17 states allow the philosophical exemption. These are Arizona, California, Colorado, Idaho, Indiana, Louisiana, Maine, Michigan, Minnesota, Nebraska, North Dakota, Ohio, Oklahoma, Utah, Vermont, Washington, and Wisconsin. (This exemption is being challenged in different states, so check this.) This is the easiest exemption to use. Parents need only state their strong personal beliefs that cause them to oppose vaccinations. As with religious exemptions, you generally will have to be opposed to all vaccinations. Some people have had their philosophical exemption requests challenged by school officials.

Your Decision

There are many questions that you should ask yourself before deciding whether or not to immunize your children. These include: (1) What is the seriousness of the disease to be immunized against? (2) Do any personal health risks exist which contraindicate a particular vaccine? (3) What are the possible side effects of the vaccine? (4) What are the risks of epidemics in my area? and (5) How does my philosophy of health and my religious convictions affect my decision? The books reviewed here should help you answer many of these questions.

You many decide to vaccinate your child according to the recommended schedule. You may decide to refuse certain vaccines based on your child's health or your concern over a particular vaccine. You may decide to delay vaccinations until your child is a little older. Or you may decide to refuse all vaccines for your child.

Remember that you do not have to make your final decision when your child is two months old. Do not let yourself be rushed into making an important decision that you are not completely comfortable with.

As you seek to do what is right for the health of your children, remember to ask for guidance and wisdom from God. This is the most important action you can take.

For those of you who are Catholic, you might wish to place your children under the protection of the Child Jesus, venerated under the title The Holy Child Jesus of Good Health (see p. 244 for information).

BOOK

REVIEWS

Using the Book Reviews

The books reviewed in this Guide represent many sides of the vaccination issue. To help you locate books of a specific kind, I have divided them into eleven and/or the books' contents. Some of the books could easily have fit into more than one section, since they cover several areas of interest. So, the sections should not be viewed as rigid divisions, but as general groupings.

Structure of the Book Reviews

All books are listed alphabetically by title within each section or subsection. If the book is indexed, footnoted, or contains a bibliography or resources, I note this.

Each book review follows the same pattern. A brief one-sentence summary of the book precedes a description of the author's background and qualifications. I explain why the book was written and for whom. Next, several paragraphs highlight the main points of the book. In some cases I include my own opinion about the contents. Remember that my conclusions and views will probably differ from yours. Obviously, I like some books more than others and it may show in the reviews. Nonetheless, I try to be as fair as possible.

The Importance of Proper Documentation

Any book on the topic of vaccination requires sound documentation for validating the author's conclusions. At the end of each book review I include a short evaluation of the author's documentation.

There are two things I evaluate in each book: (1) the use or non-use of footnotes; and (2) the type of sources used. Some books are easier to critique in this regard than others. For example, some books have no footnotes at all. Others have a few. And still others are drowning in quote after quote.

The most important question is whether or not the authors correctly evaluate, quote, or interpret their sources or whether they distort them, take them out of context, or simply misunderstand them. Unfortunately, such in-depth critique is mostly beyond the scope of a collection of reviews such as this one. However, where I am aware of any problems with sources, I will state it in the review.

A book with a sloppy bibliography, poor use of references, or inaccurate information casts doubt upon the quality of the author's research and the author's conclusions. With a topic as controversial as vaccination, meticulous attention to detail lends credibility to the whole book.

Documentation of the Books Reviewed

Many of the authors critical of vaccination tend to rely on consumer health books, or other general books on vaccination for source material. In place of hard data, some authors use strong emotional language to convince the reader. Emotion is fine as long as the author has evidence to back up claims.

On the other hand, most of the pro-vaccination books contain large bibliographies composed almost solely of medical journal articles. I can not judge the quality of the work of the scientists performing the research or writing the report in the medical journals. Again, you run into the question of whether data is taken out of context, etc. The dry, technical language of many of these books lends an authoritative voice to them and a false impression of disinterest and non-bias. The lack of emotion and heavy use of statistical data effectively eliminates the human element from the discussion and neglects the question of ethics.

Some authors rely on individual case histories, e.g., reports by parents about their children's reactions to vaccines. These I consider important primary sources. Unfortunately, most pro-vaccination authors disregard these as anecdotal and statistically invalid (too many variables, no controls, etc.). I find it unfortunate that physicians' experiences "on the front lines" are not considered to be scientifically valid.

Some of these books contain unsubstantiated material, not because the author was sloppy, but because no scientific data exists. They only have the experiences and hunches of doctors and parents to go on. If an author states up front that his ideas are speculative or that there is not sufficient evidence to make any hard claims and uses his book as a spring board to encourage further research, that's entirely different from the author who claims to have all the facts, but has no proof in his pockets.

Research Practices

There are several research practices that I've noticed that disturb me. One is the practice by some authors critical of vaccinations of quoting from other authors who have also written books critical of vaccinations. There is nothing wrong with this, per se, however, it removes the second authors one step farther away from the original source material. Maybe I've read too many of these books, but sometimes I get the feeling that everybody is just quoting everybody else. Of course, this doesn't apply to all authors reviewed here. However, in some instances when one author quotes heavily from another author, I wonder if the second author doesn't just end up with his or her book being a paraphrase of the first author. I think you get the point.

The second practice that I don't like much is when one author quotes a source that was quoted in another author's book. As long as the second author mentions in the text that this quote actually appeared in someone else's book, thus alerting the reader that the second author did not actually read the original source, that's okay. But, if the second author "buries" this fact in the footnote, then the reader who doesn't bother to read footnotes will not realize the truth about where this quote came from. It is certainly a better research practice for the second author to have read the document in which the quote originally appeared to make sure that the first author actually quoted the source accurately. Of course, if the original source is no longer available or very difficult to obtain, that's another matter.

In this case, the second author should simply state the situation in the text, instead of burying it in the footnote.

A worse practice which follows from the above, is if an author quotes a source quoted by another author, but instead of indicating in the text or footnote that the quote came via this other author's book, just lists the original citation from the first author. This leads the reader to assume that the second author read the original document, when this is not actually the case. Obviously, I can't tell if an author does this, but sometimes I wonder.

If You Want to Read the Whole Book

Once you decide which books you'd like to read in full, you can make a trip to your local library and find many of them, or if not, you can request them through interlibrary loan. If you wish to purchase any, I list after each book review under the heading "Available From", the name of publisher, or any organizations that sells that book. Each listing is followed by a number in parentheses. This number refers to the numbered section in Resources where that company or organization is listed.

Section A

Introductory Books

Section A.1: Books for Parents

The books reviewed in this section are books written specifically for parents who are beginning their research into vaccinations. The authors want to help parents make an informed decision. Most of the authors systematically address each of the childhood diseases and vaccines along with the risks and benefits of the vaccines. Some authors add information on the history of vaccination. Some discuss the immune system and how vaccines work. Most of the authors provide information about mandatory vaccination laws and obtaining legal exemptions.

Many of these authors are personally opposed to vaccinations, however, they try to present balanced information and encourage readers to make their own decision.

The Consumer's Guide to Childhood Vaccines
Barbara Loe Fisher. Vienna, VA: National Vaccine Information Center. 1997. 89 pp. ISBN 1-889204-01-3. Glossary. Bibliography.

This guide for parents is written by Barbara Loe Fisher, co-founder of the National Vaccine Information Center (NVIC). This book is a summary for parents of basic information on childhood vaccines with an emphasis on how to prevent vaccine injury.

Ms. Fisher describes in detail all of the "vaccine-preventable" childhood diseases. There are chapters on each vaccine, including reactions and how to report them. Contraindications are listed. She also notes the narrowing of absolute contraindications and possible contraindications. She gives explicit information on what to do before your child is vaccinated to help lower the possibility that your child will suffer a vaccine injury. For example, make sure your child isn't sick that day, request the vaccine package insert (preferably beforehand), explain any possible contraindications or health conditions you are concerned about, and make sure the vaccine lot number is recorded in your child's records. Legal exemptions are also covered. Ms. Fisher lists several alternative health organizations for readers to contact if they are interested in other health care treatments for childhood diseases or treating the effects of vaccine damage.

Ms. Fisher is careful to use material mainly from government medical reports (e.g., CDC, IOM), medical journals, and vaccine product inserts for her sources. This is especially true when she presents evidence showing causality for various adverse effects and diseases from vaccines, and when she lists accepted contraindications. A very helpful glossary explains medical terms used to describe various adverse reactions. The book is not footnoted, although the sources Ms. Fisher used are listed in the bibliography. While this may make it more difficult for readers to check her sources, much of it can easily be verified by logging onto the CDC website (www.cdc.gov/nip).

Ms. Fisher succinctly states the basic facts that parents need who are first confronting this issue. She clearly presents accurate, reliable information.

Available From:
Koren Publications (8). NVIC (1).

Parents Guide to Childhood Immunizations
Centers for Disease Control and Prevention. Atlanta, GA: U.S. Dept. of Health and Human Services. 1993. 39 pp.

This booklet describes all the universally recommended childhood vaccines. It is updated periodically. As expected, the seriousness of each disease is stressed. There is a one-page overview of what antibodies are and how vaccines create them. The authors admit that adverse reactions sometimes occur and that some people should not receive certain vaccines because of health condition.

They minimize the seriousness of adverse reactions that have been associated with the DPT vaccine. For example, for a child who had convulsions after a DPT shot, it states that the fever after the shot caused the convulsions, not the vaccine. And fever-related convulsions as "one expert" they state believes, do not cause permanent damage.

In the introduction, it states that parents should make an informed decision, but it adds that vaccinations are mandatory and your child should be "protected". Gone is the oft quoted line from the 1979 edition: "The decision to have your child vaccinated is yours, alone, to make."

At the end of each chapter is a paragraph summarizing state laws for that particular vaccine. No mention of legal exemptions is made, and no mention is made of how to report adverse reactions to VAERS, nor is information presented about the National Vaccine Injury Compensation Program. Parents are merely told to notify their doctor if any "serious problems" arise. This book contains no references or bibliography.

Available From:
National Immunization Program (1). Free.

Vaccine Choices, Homeopathic Alternatives and Parental Rights: A Sourcepack of Information for Healthcare Consumers and Concerned Parents
Patty Brennan. Michigan: The Holistic Midwifery Institute. 1997. 42 pp. Report. Appendices. Catalogs.

This sourcepack was written and compiled by Patty Brennan, a midwife in Michigan. She conducts workshops on vaccinations, childcare, and homeopathy. She initially wrote it for use by her students, but it is of use for anyone first approaching this subject and especially so, Michigan residents.

She presents an overview of each of the universally recom-mended childhood vaccines and includes information on the history of each vaccine. She lists ways to support and strengthen the immune system such as breastfeeding, avoiding the overuse of antibiotics, and better nutrition, among other things. She includes books she recommends for further reading.

She discusses homeopathy and vaccination in great detail which is why I almost chose to list this sourcepack in the Homeopathy Section. She gives dosage information for using homeopathic remedies for vaccine adverse reactions. This is something I have not seen before. She also lists homeopathic remedies for prevention and treatment of childhood diseases. In fact, she uses Susan Curtis' book, *A Handbook of Homeopathic Alternatives to Immunisation*, and Leslie Speight's book, *Homeopathy and Immunization*, as references (both are reviewed in Section I). Ms. Brennan also refers to Dr. Isaac Golden and his development of homeopathic vaccines. She lists a sample chart showing the remedy and age of administration for people who may be interested in this method. She refers readers to Dr. Golden's book, *Vaccination? A Review of Risks and Alternatives*, for more details. (See review in Section I).

Ms. Brennan's sourcepack includes an appendix that contains among other things: (1) current copies of the CDC's Vaccine Information Statements (reviewed in this Section); (2) a VAERS report form; (3) a list of foods which boost the immune system; (4) Michigan immunization laws and waiver form; (5) information on several vaccine organizations; and (6) vaccine book catalogs.

Ms. Brennan's sourcepack is a concise introduction for parents who are new to this issue. She collects together a lot of valuable vaccine-related materials for easy of use by all.

Available From:
The Holistic Midwifery Institute (2).

Vaccination: Examining the Record
Judith A. DeCava, BS, CNC. Columbus, GA: Brentwood Academic Press. 1994. 119 pp. No ISBN. Bibliography.

This book examines whether vaccines work, are effective, or safe. Judith DeCava is a certified Nutritional Consultant having served with various physicians over the past 16 years. She is also a writer for the National Academy of Research Biochemists and executive vice president of the Biomedical Health Foundation.

This book is similar in structure to the other books reviewed in this Section. Ms. DeCava devotes half the book to examining vaccinations in general and the other half to each vaccine separately.

She includes a chapter describing how the immune system works and another on "immune theory", i.e., the germ theory of disease. From the tone of her writing, she is quite skeptical of the germ theory.

She has an interesting chapter describing bacteria and viruses in which she presents information from various medical textbooks, which show the problems surrounding what viruses, actually are. We know viruses are a strand of DNA or RNA wrapped in a protein coat, but, she states, it is not known whether they are alive or not, or how they actually function in our cells. She describes how cells are prepared to be seen by an electron microscope. This preparation consists of cutting cells into thin slices and staining them with chemical compounds. The cells are not alive or whole when they are viewed, which obviously affects what can be seen and understood about cellular activity using these microscopes.

In another chapter, she explains what vaccines contain and whether they are safe and effective. She includes lots of quotes from other general vaccination books to support her view that vaccines are not safe (e.g., from *What About Immunizations* by C. Cournoyer, see review in this Section, and *Immunizations: The Reality Behind the Myth* by W. James, reviewed in Section C). Her description of what vaccines contain lumps ingredients of all vaccines together, which makes it unclear which vaccines contain which substances.

A chapter on possible long-term neurological damage is derived heavily from Harris Coulter's book, *Vaccination, Social Violence and Criminality* (reviewed in Section B.2).

The individual chapters on vaccines include ones on DPT, MMR, polio, Hib, hepatitis B, influenza, smallpox, and pneumonia vaccines. She briefly describes each disease and vaccine, mentions statistics which state that disease incidence was falling long before vaccination was introduced, describes adverse reactions, and gives examples of vaccine failure (i.e., percentages of children catching the disease they were vaccinated against).

I note one important error: She incorrectly quotes from Neil Miller's book, *Vaccines: Are They Really Safe and Effective?* (reviewed in this Section) that the conjugated Hib vaccine is derived from human blood products. This is not true. Another vaccine is being investigated, according to Mr. Miller, possibly using human blood products, but the current conjugated Hib vaccines do not contain any human blood products.

Overall, this is a useful introductory book, especially for the information Ms. DeCava provides questioning vaccine safety and effectiveness. It is footnoted with articles from medical journals, medical textbooks, and consumer vaccination books.

Available From:
In the National Health Federation's "Immunization Kit" (See Section B.1).

The Vaccine Guide: Making an Informed Choice
Randall Neustaedter, OMD. Berkeley, CA: North Atlantic Books and Homeopathic Educational Services. 1996. 260 pp. ISBN 1-55643-215-1. Index. Bibliography. Resources.
(An earlier edition was published under the title *The Immunization Decision*, and prior to that edition it was published as *Immunizations: Are They Necessary?*)

This is the new edition of Dr. Neustaedter's previous book, *The Immunization Decision*. It is over twice the length of this earlier book. As the subtitle states, Dr. Neustaedter helps parents make an informed choice regarding vaccinations for their children. Dr. Neustaedter is a homeopathic practitioner specializing in child health care with a doctorate in Oriental Medicine. His philosophy of health is in direct opposition to the theory upon which vaccination is based, but he does not let this overly influence his desire to let parents decide for themselves, and he maintains an even-handed and balanced approach throughout the book.

Dr. Neustaedter expanded the section on deciding if, when, and which vaccines to give your child, incorporating more medical references and a lengthier look at alternative health systems, especially homeopathy. He stresses that parents can become informed enough about vaccines to make a decision regarding their use that they will feel comfortable with. He helps parents by addressing the questions most parents have about vaccines: short and long-term adverse reactions and the timing and choosing of vaccines.

This latter point — determining when to give your child a particular vaccine and deciding whether to refuse certain ones — is not discussed much by other authors. Other authors, who oppose vaccinations on philosophical grounds, or on the grounds of short and long-term adverse reactions, tend to dismiss the use of all vaccines. By telling parents that they can delay shots until the child is older, or refuse only certain ones, Dr. Neustaedter is going beyond the "yes" or "no" decision which parents may feel they must make, and instead he helps them realize that their decision can be a combination of both "yes" and "no" and "we'll wait awhile".

He also examines the ingredients in vaccines and adverse reactions associated with these ingredients. He includes a chapter critiquing conventional vaccine studies. He shows how case studies can be flawed in design and distort results. He asserts that and those running a study are in many cases affiliated with vaccine manufacturers.

He includes a whole chapter on homeopathic vaccines and quotes the work of Isaac Golden, DC (see review of his work in Section I) in this regard. He presents the history of homeopathic vaccines and studies that indicate their safety and effectiveness, but he is quick to add that no long-term studies have been conducted to evaluate the lasting effectiveness of homeopathic vaccines used for prevention (rather than for treatment of the disease) though some practitioners (e.g., Golden) feel that they are effective.

He briefly presents factors that affect our immune system that we have direct control over regarding our children's health. These are: (1) breastfeeding; (2) good nutrition; (3) adequate sanitation and hygienic living conditions; and (4) environment that supports the mental and emotional health of our children.

He explains legal exemptions and quotes from various court cases, especially concerning religious exemptions, which support a parents' right to seek a legal exemption.

In the second half of the book he describes the following vaccines in individual chapters: tetanus, polio, pertussis, acellular pertussis, diphtheria, measles, mumps, rubella, Hib, hepatitis B, chickenpox, and pneumococcal vaccine. For each of these he gives a summary of the disease and development of the vaccine, looks at vaccine effectiveness, and describes short and long-term adverse reactions. He quotes from medical studies throughout and includes relevant statistics whenever possible. At the end of each chapter he presents his own recommendations about that particular vaccine, while making it clear that it is up to the parents to make any final decisions.

Dr. Neustaedter has written a thorough, balanced introductory book on immunizations which covers many areas of controversy regarding the safety and effectiveness of vaccines and accomplishes his stated goal of helping parents make an informed choice. It is well-footnoted and researched with medical journal articles.

Available From:
American Vegan Society (2). Homeopathic Educational Services (2). New Atlantean Press (8). Koren Publications (8). NVIC (1). The Minimum Price Homeopathic Books (8). North Atlantic Books (8).

Vaccine Information Statements:
"Diphtheria, Tetanus, and Pertussis Vaccine (DTP)". 1991: 11 pp. 1994 and after: 2 pp. Current edition: 8/97.
"Measles, Mumps, and Rubella Vaccine (MMR)". 1991: 10 pp. 1994 and after: 2 pp. Current edition: 12/98.
"Polio Vaccine". 1991: 10 pp. 1994 and after: 2 pp. Current edition: 1/2000.
"Tetanus and Diphtheria Vaccine (Td)". 1991: 8 pp. 1994 current edition: 2 pp.
"Hepatitis B Vaccine". 1998: 2 pp.
"*Haemophilus* Influenzae type b Vaccine (Hib)". 1998: 2 pp.
"Chickenpox Vaccine". 1998: 2 pp.
Centers for Disease Control and Prevention (CDC). The 1991 editions are called Vaccine Information Pamphlets" (VIPs). The 1994 and later editions are called "Vaccine Information Statements" (VISs).

The National Childhood Vaccine Injury Act of 1986 (NCVIA) mandated that Vaccine Information Pamphlets (VIPs) be created to inform parents of the risks and benefits for each of the then univer-sally recommended childhood vaccines. The VIPs were published in 1991. In 1994 new VIPs, now called Vaccine Information State-ments (VISs) were issued. In August 1997, Hib, hepatitis B, and chickenpox were added to the Vaccine Injury Compensation System and VISs were issued for them as well. Below are descriptions of the 1991 versions (VIPs), followed by description of the 1994 versions (VISs) to show you the differences between the two.

Each of the VIPs contained: (1) a description of the disease; (2) a discussion of possible adverse reactions from the vaccine; (3) confirmation that the benefits outweigh the risks; (4) the recommended schedule of doses; (5) a list of who should not receive the shot or should have the shot delayed; (6) information on monitoring your child for a reaction after the shot; and (7) how to report any adverse reactions. The last page of each VIP contained a Vaccine Administration Record for use by the doctor in filling out all the legally required information about the vaccine given. This required information includes the vaccine manufacturer, lot number, and name and address of the health care provider giving the shot. The VIPs stressed the importance of vaccinations and minimized any risks. An important feature was the list of contraindications and the adverse reaction reporting information.

In 1993, the Department of Health and Human Services successfully lobbied Congress to amend the NCVIA to discontinue use of the VIPs on the grounds that they were an impediment to immunization because they were too long and hard to read. The VIPs have been replaced, as of October 1, 1994, by two-sided flyers called Vaccine Information Statements (VISs). To aid in reading comprehension, the reading level of the VISs has been lowered from an 8th grade reading level used in all the VIPs, to 5th to 7th grade reading levels (boy, Johnny really can't read!).

The VISs contain a concise description of the benefits of the vaccine and a concise description of the risks. Contraindications are listed, but are not named as such. The VISs just state that you should inform your doctor if the person to be vaccinated has certain health conditions without specifically stating that you should not receive a particular vaccine because of these conditions. (Read the CDC's *Guide to Contraindications to Childhood Vaccinations* reviewed in Section B.1 for more details). However, at least the phone number of the National Vaccine Injury Compensation Program is still listed. As of October 1, 1994, health care providers are no longer required by federal law to obtain the signature of the parent or guardian to acknowledge receipt of the VISs, as was required previously for the VIPs, though some states still require it.

Please note, as CDC recommendations change the VISs are updated. Most notably the Polio VIS was updated in January 2000 when an all IPV polio schedule was recommended.

Available From:
National Immunization Program (1). Free.

Vaccines: Are They Really Safe and Effective?

Neil Z. Miller. Santa Fe, NM: New Atlantean Press. Revised. 1999. 78 pp. ISBN 1-881217-10-8. Endnotes.

For those of you without a lot of time, this book presents many of the concerns that other authors address, but in an abbreviated form. Neil Miller is a research journalist and natural health advocate. The revised 1999 edition contains minor changes and updates from the 1996 edition (but not enough changes to affect the number of pages or the ISBN number).

Mr. Miller briefly describes each childhood disease and corresponding vaccine. He includes Hib and hepatitis B, but not chicken pox. His conclusions are that vaccines do not work and they cause many adverse reactions. There is a chapter on possible long-term adverse effects of vaccines such as immune system malfunctions (e.g., autoimmune diseases or cancers), developmental delays, autism, and other learning disorders. He also discusses vaccine contraindications at length. The National Childhood Vaccine Injury Act of 1986, which set up a compensation system for vaccine-damaged children, is explained in detail. He also briefly disputes the germ theory.

It is a good "first book", because it is well footnoted enabling you to easily research any topic that interests you. His references are from medical journals, medical textbooks, government reports, consumer health magazines, and consumer books on vaccination.

Available From:
American Vegan Society (2). Global Vaccine Awareness League (1). Koren Publications (8). The Minimum Price Homeopathic Books (8). Natural Hygiene, Inc. (2). NVIC (1). Nelson's Books (8). New Atlantean Press (8). Also available at bookstores nationwide.

What About Immunizations? Exposing the Vaccine Philosophy
Cynthia Cournoyer. Santa Cruz, CA: Nelson's Books. 6th Edition. 1995.
207 pp. ISBN 0-9612188-5-1. Endnotes. Resources.

Cynthia Cournoyer defines what she coined the "vaccine philosophy" as the belief that vaccines are safe and effective and any risks are far outweighed by the benefits. This is certainly the sentiment of the medical community and it is what we have been told to believe all our lives. In this book, Ms. Cournoyer presents evidence to cast doubt on this theory. Ms. Cournoyer is a mother and has researched vaccinations for 13 years. She approaches the topic from the perspective of a concerned parent.

In the first part of this book, she casts doubt upon the germ theory of disease and supports the views that the condition of the body is the principal factor in disease, not the presence of germs (see Section C for more information about this view). She includes a chapter on how vaccines appear to work and one on what vaccines do to our bodies. She concludes that they do not effectively confer immunity and they may even cause unknown, long-term ill effects.

In the second part of the book she explains in separate chapters each of the usual childhood vaccines (including acellular pertussis, chickenpox, and hepatitis B) and the adverse reactions associated with the vaccines.

New to the sixth edition is a chapter on how vaccine practices are continued, which looks at the medical machinery behind our vaccine policies and beliefs. She also discusses legal exemptions.

What makes this book unique is her many quotes from parents sharing their feelings about their experiences with vaccination, especially regarding the decision they have made and pressures they encountered to vaccinate.

Ms. Cournoyer's book is well footnoted and documented. Her sources are other consumer vaccination books (many reviewed here) and medical journals. Her book is easy to read, summarizes the prevailing arguments against vaccination, and provides counsel and encouragement to parents trying to make an informed decision.

Available From:
Out of print.

What Every Parent Should Know About Childhood Immunization

Jamie Murphy. Boston: Earth Healing Products. 1993. 192 pp.
ISBN 0-9630373-0-7. Index. Endnotes.

If you are looking for a good, well written introductory book on vaccination this is an excellent choice. Mr. Murphy is a writer with a long-term interest in natural health and vaccination.

This book begins with a chapter describing the immune system and another comparing artificially acquired immunity to naturally acquired immunity. Mr. Murphy is concerned with the possibility of the viruses from vaccines "hiding" in cells and later in life being "triggered" to become cancer or other autoimmune diseases. He does not reject immunization by rejecting the germ theory, but instead critiques the mechanism of how immunization works against accepted medical theories and uses medical source material.

Mr. Murphy includes detailed chapters on how vaccines are made and the toxic chemicals of which they are composed. For those of you concerned about animal rights, there is a chapter on animal experimentation in vaccine development. I applaud Mr. Murphy for including a chapter on breast milk, explaining its vital importance in building an infant's immune system. (I have written several editions of my book, including this one, with a nursing baby on my lap.) He has separate chapters on whooping cough (pertussis) and the 1980's outbreak of measles; otherwise, he does not examine individual vaccines. (You will need to read other books for information on each childhood disease and vaccine.) There is a chapter presenting the history of mandatory vaccination laws and a lengthy chapter describing how to obtain legal exemptions from these laws. He even explains several state laws in detail. The information contained in this chapter is very extensive.

One major mistake must be noted, however; on page 26 he indicates that MMR is a killed virus vaccine. This is wrong. It is a live virus vaccine.

This book is well documented and footnoted throughout with medical journal and medical textbook sources. His book is a welcome addition to the continuing debate over vaccination.

Available From:
American Vegan Society (2). Earth Healing Products (8). ICEA (2). Koren Publications (8). NVIC (1). Nelson's Books (8).

What Every Parent Should Know About Vaccines
Paul A. Offit, M.D. and Louis M. Bell, M.D. New York, NY: Macmillan Publishing USA. 1998. 226 pp. ISBN 0-02-862009-7. References. Index. (A new edition has come out in January 2000. The title has been changed to *Vaccines: What Every Parent Should Know.*)

This book clearly presents basic information about childhood diseases and vaccines for them. Dr. Paul Offit is chief of the Section of Infectious Disease at the Children's Hospital of Philadelphia. Dr. Louis Bell is an attending physician in the Section of Infectious Disease and the Section of Emergency Medicine at the Children's Hospital of Philadelphia. Both are also Associate Professors of Pediatrics at the University of Pennsylvania School of Medicine. They strongly advocate the use of vaccines. The book is well laid out. It is apparent from the tone of the introduction, that the authors wish to reassure parents, who may have read alarmist news reports or books, that vaccines are safe and still needed.

The authors divide the book into five parts. Part I contains chapters on how vaccines are made, how they work, whether they are safe, and who recommends them. The chapter on how vaccines are made is fantastic. They take complex procedures and explain them simply, plainly, and accurately. The reader is clearly aware of the difference between a killed bacterial vaccine and a live, weakened virus vaccine. Unfortunately, some of the authors who have written books critical of vaccines do a poor job of explaining how vaccines are made. Many of these books contain errors, outdated information, or vague statements. Drs. Offit and Bell offer one of the clearest explanations for the lay reader of how vaccines are made that I've read.

Part II of the book covers vaccines recommended for all children. The authors cover each childhood disease and vaccine. They provide even further detailed information in these chapters on how each of these vaccines are made and how they differ or are similar to each other. The vaccines covered are DTaP, Polio, Hib, MMR,

Hepatitis B, and varicella (chickenpox). The authors severely down-play any adverse reactions. They constantly repeat that nobody died from such-and-such vaccine, but people have died from the disease. They stress that serious side effects are rare and hardly worth con-sidering. Even the problems with the whole-cell, killed pertussis vaccine are downplayed. The authors list few contraindications to vaccines.

The authors include a chapter on "vaccine myths". Some of the "myths" really do appear to be myths (e.g., "vaccines don't work"). But other "myths" are not so easily dismissed. For example, "vaccines weaken the immune system". To refute this myth, the authors explain the research of Dr. Mel Cohn and Dr. Rodney Langman of The Salk Institute in San Diego who think it depends upon your size how many microorganisms you can respond to. They estimate, for example, that elephant's immune systems can respond to 100 times as many microorganisms as humans. They estimate that humans can respond to about 100,000 different organisms. So, conclude Drs. Offit and Bell, only 0.01% of the immune system is used up by children responding to the ten childhood vaccines. These authors do not mention the difference in size between an adult and a child nor the fact that an infant's immune system is not completely developed. I find this quite interesting. I thought the idea that the immune system could be used up at all was a wild idea. I did not know that it was a serious theory. The authors do not state that unknown long-term adverse effects are a myth; they do not discuss this at all.

Part III of the book covers vaccines for children who are high risk for that disease. These diseases are rabies, influenza, pneumococcus, meningococcus and tuberculosis. You may have heard news stories about outbreaks of meningitis among college students and that the meningococcal vaccine has been recommended for college freshmen. The authors state that there are at least five different types of meningococcus. The current vaccine only contains four of these five types. The type B meningococcus is very hard to make antibodies against, and researchers have been unable to make it into a vaccine. Unfortunately, the authors state, fifty percent of meningococcal cases are caused by type B. The vaccine can do nothing to prevent infection from type B. The CDC announced on October 21, 1999 that it was recommending the vaccine for college freshman. The CDC said that statistics from 1998-1999 showed that 70% of the meningitis cases from college students were types "C" or "Y", which are contained in the vaccine.

Part IV of the book covers vaccines for children traveling abroad. This section makes the crucial distinction between "required" and "recommended" vaccines. The authors state that most people assume that if a vaccine is required for entry to a certain country that there must be a strong chance of exposure to that disease, and if a vaccine is only recommended, that there must be little chance for exposure to that disease. Actually, as the authors explain, the opposite is true. Countries require visitors to have certain vaccines to keep those diseases out of their country. Vaccines are recommended for visitors going to countries or certain areas within a country that have outbreaks of that disease. So, you are more likely to be exposed to a disease for which a vaccine is recommended, not required. The diseases they cover in this section are hepatitis A, cholera, typhoid, yellow fever, and Japanese Encephalitis Virus. As with the other vaccines covered in this book, the authors explain how they are made, how effective they are, and who should get them.

Part V of the book covers vaccines for the near future. One of these vaccines is for rotavirus. This book was written prior to the release of the rotavirus vaccine in August 1998, but it was in clinical trials at the time and the authors had access to this information. They state that the vaccine is safe. They do not even qualify their statement with something like "so far clinical trials indicate the vaccine is safe". They just state that the vaccine is safe. Well, as we all know, the vaccine was not safe and was recalled by the manufacturer in October 1999. The other vaccines they discuss are ones for Lyme disease and Respiratory Syncytial virus (viral pneumonia vaccine).

Overall, this book is a well-written, accurate, introductory text for parents. The authors excel in clearly explaining how each vaccine is made, something few other authors writing for a lay audience accomplish accurately. Their weakness is their brushing over adverse reactions and downplaying contraindications. I would recommend that readers combine this book with another that covers these areas in more detail, for example, *The Consumer's Guide to Childhood Vaccines*, by NVIC, also reviewed in this Section.

   The book is not footnoted, however the authors do include a list of the references they used for each chapter. Their material is almost solely from government reports, medical textbooks, and medical journals.

Available From:
IDG Books (8). Bookstores nationwide.

Section A.2

Infant Health Care Books

There are quite a number of books on childcare and infant health that contain chapters on vaccinations. I have included a few here. The ones I have chosen to include give extensive coverage to immunizations and as you will quickly see, tend to be skeptical of routine vaccinations and are opposed to mandatory vaccination laws. In the "unrandom" survey I made of infant care books at my local library, I found that most authors cover the topic of immunizations in at best several pages and at worst a paragraph or two. Generally, the information is limited to explaining the diseases for which vaccines are recommended and stating how important they are in disease prevention. Dr. William Sears in his book, *The Baby Book*, does go into some detail on short-term adverse reactions, but he was an exception among the pile of books I examined.

Everywoman's Book
Paavo Airola. Sherwood, OR: Health Plus Publishers. 1979. 640 pp.
ISBN 0-932090-10-9. Index. Endnotes.

This book is on women's and infant health. Paavo Airola is a nutritionist and authority on biological medicine. He has published many books on holistic health.

Contained in this book is a 23-page chapter on vaccination. Dr. Airola opposes vaccinations by refuting the germ theory of disease. He believes that disease occurs only when the body is out of balance with itself. Germs alone do not cause disease. He is in favor of improving the immune system naturally by taking vitamin C during an infection, and eating lactic acid fermented foods (yogurt, pickled vegetables, and sourdough bread) to promote the production of lactic acid producing bacteria in the intestines, which aid the body to fight infection. If you chose to vaccinate your children, he advises giving them large doses of vitamin C concurrently to help aid their body in handling the vaccination.

He advises parents to make a studied decision. He views tetanus vaccine as having the least adverse effects of the available vaccines. (He wrote this before Hib, hepatitis B, and chickenpox vaccines were available). He is opposed to mandatory vaccination.

He footnotes his book with research from medical journals and other general health books, including alternative health books.

Available From:
Out of print.

How to Raise a Healthy Child. . . In Spite of Your Doctor

Robert S. Mendelsohn, M.D. NY: Ballantine Books. 1984. 283 pp. ISBN 0-345-34276-3. Index. Bibliography.

This book is primarily medical advice for new parents. The late Dr. Mendelsohn, a pediatrician for 30 years, criticizes many of the established medical practices of pediatricians. This includes vaccination.

He discusses vaccinations for twenty pages. He lists all the childhood vaccines in use in 1984 (Hib, hepatitis B, and chickenpox are not included) and why he opposes them. This is a summary of his ideas presented in "The People's Doctor" newsletters compiled in book form in *Immunizations: The Terrible Risks Your Children Face that Your Doctor Won't Reveal* (reviewed in Section B.1).

This is a mass market paperback and may still be available in bookstores. There is no documentation or references cited.

Available From:
American Vegan Society (1). Koren Publications (8). National Health Federation (2). New Atlantean Press (8). Random House, Inc. (8).

**Take Charge of Your Child's Health: A Guide to Recognizing
Symptoms and Treating Minor Illnesses at Home**
George Wootan, M.D. and Sarah Verney. NY: Crown Publishing. 1992.
350 pp. ISBN 0-517-57365-2. Index. Endnotes. Bibliography.
This book was issued in a second edition in January 2000. NY: Marlowe &
Co. 388 pp. ISBN 1-56924653-X.

This book contains practical advice for keeping your baby healthy
naturally, without overdue dependence on medicine and doctors.
George Wootan is a family practitioner and medical advisor for La
Leche League. Susan Verney is a freelance writer.

One chapter in this book is devoted to the topic of vaccination
(40 pages). Dr. Wootan briefly describes childhood diseases and
vaccines. He argues that most infectious diseases were declining in
incidence long before vaccinations began and therefore vaccines can
not take all the credit. He covers adverse reactions and contraindications and gives his personal opinion about whether or not your child
should receive a particular vaccine. Overall, he only recommends
the tetanus vaccine (for the same reasons as Neustaedter in his book
The Vaccine Guide reviewed in Section A.1) believing that the
others either have too many adverse reactions (pertussis), have
outlived their usefulness (diphtheria and polio), or have question-
able efficacy (MMR). He briefly expresses caution about accepting
new vaccines whose long-term ill effects have yet to be determined.
Although he does give his own recommendations, he stresses that
parents should make their own decision based on their "faith
system".

Each chapter is footnoted. He lists recommended books for
additional reading. I highly recommend it as a source book of practical information to aid you in taking care of your children's health.

Available From:
The 1992 edition is out of print. The 2000 edition is distributed by
Publishers Group West (8).

Section B

Vaccine Safety and Effectiveness

This section is divided into four parts. Part 1 covers short and long-term adverse reactions associated with a variety of childhood vaccines. Part 2 examines the whole-cell, killed pertussis component of the DTP vaccine. This vaccine has now been replaced by the safer acellular pertussis vaccine. Part 3 contains books that explore how vaccines affect the immune system in general. Part 4 briefly explains the current concerns with the MMR and hepatitis B vaccines.

Section B.1: Short and Long-term Adverse Reactions

Unlike the authors in Section A, who present an overview of vaccination, the authors in this section focus on the possible adverse effects of vaccines. Some discuss only short-term reactions such as immediate neurological damage. Others are concerned about the possibility of unknown long-term adverse effects. Still others look at historical vaccine mishaps. Three of the books below are staunchly pro-vaccination, but the authors agree that the risks associated with vaccines must be acknowledged to prevent future problems.

Adverse Events Associated with Childhood Vaccines: Evidence Bearing on Causality
Kathleen R. Stratton, Cynthia J. Howe, and Richard B. Johnston, Jr., eds. Vaccine Safety Committee, Division of Health Promotion and Disease Prevention, Institute of Medicine. Washington, D.C.: National Academy Press. 1994. 464 pp. ISBN 0-309-04895-8. Index. Bibliography. Endnotes. Glossary.

This book is the report by the Vaccine Safety Committee of its review of all available literature on adverse events associated with childhood vaccines. This report was mandated by Section 313 of the National Childhood Vaccine Injury Act of 1986 (NCVIA).

The Vaccine Safety Committee, composed of 14 members, worked on this report for 18 months. The members are professionals (mostly medical professors) from the fields of immunology, pediatrics, internal medicine, infectious diseases, neurology, virology, microbiology, epidemiology, and public health. The committee met six times over the course of 18 months. They reviewed 7000 abstracts of scientific and medical studies and read 2000 books and articles. They held two public meetings where parents and other interested parties (e.g., NVIC) presented evidence. Two scientific meetings open only to invited scientists were also held. It is obvious that the committee members reviewed an enormous amount of material — the largest overview of the subject that I have seen.

The authors present a much more detailed explanation of the meaning of causality and the research methods they used for determining causality, than was presented in the first study mandated by the NCVIA, *Adverse Events Associated with Pertussis and Rubella Vaccines* (see review in Section B.2). This report does not repeat the work of this earlier committee; hence, it contains information on all current universally recommended childhood vaccines except pertussis and rubella (or the newer ones).

The committee included case studies and observations from parents and doctors in its report, although its main focus is on statistical analyses. (A basic understanding of statistics would be helpful.) The language is pretty sterile, but not overly technical.

The committee members considered specific adverse events and then attempted to determine if a particular vaccine may have caused that event. For two-thirds(!) of the adverse events that they considered they found insufficient data to establish or reject causality. This was due to either lack of data or an abundance of data that did not clearly show cause or lack of cause. What does this tell me? It tells me that much more research needs to be done on vaccine safety.

I will summarize the few adverse events for which they found evidence of causality: (1) anaphylaxis (a system-wide allergic reaction to a vaccine causing among other symptoms, hives, seizures, collapse, or even death) due to DT/Td/T, MMR and hepatitis B vaccines; (2) contracting polio from oral polio vaccine; and (3) Guillain-Barre syndrome related to DT/Td/T and OPV vaccines. (This disease is discussed at length.)

The Vaccine Adverse Event Reporting System (VAERS) is explained. This system was established in November 1990. Certain adverse events occurring after vaccination and within specified time frames require mandatory reporting. However, because it is a passive reporting system there is no way to know if a doctor fails to report a notifiable adverse event. The authors admit that prior to VAERS, reporting of adverse events was very low, but has increased some since VAERS started. After analyzing many of the reports, the committee found that most did not contain enough information to establish causality. (Therefore, keep good records of your child's shots and detailed accounts of any reactions, so you'll be prepared if you need to report anything to VAERS).

They also note that little research has been done to monitor the effects of multiple vaccinations upon the body (e.g., polio, DPT, Hib and now, hepatitis B, all given at the same visit).

This is the most extensive review of the literature on adverse events that has been conducted as of 1994. Being pro-vaccination scientists, the committee members are not hasty in making any conclusions. It's especially valuable to read how they did their research and evaluation of the materials. The bibliography alone is 100 pages long!

Available From:
National Academy Press (8).

Guide to Contraindications to Childhood Vaccinations
The National Immunization Program. Atlanta, GA: Centers for Disease
Control and Prevention (CDC). 21 pp.

This booklet contains the current recommendations of the Advisory
Committee on Immunization (ACIP) and the Committee on Infec-
tious Diseases (Red Book committee) of the American Academy of
Pediatrics (AAP) both of whom routinely publish recommendations
regarding childhood immunizations. It is updated periodically.
(ACIP recommendations are available free from the CDC National
Immunization Program, see Vaccination Organizations in Resources. The Red Book committee publishes their recommendations
in *The Report of the Committee on Infectious Diseases*, reviewed in
Section E.)
    This booklet lists valid and not valid contraindications to each
of the following universally recommended childhood vaccines.
Your healthcare provider can use this guide to screen patients who
should not receive particular vaccines because of certain health
conditions. It's set up in chart format with "yes" and "no" columns
and a few "special notes" making it easy for anyone to use.
    The preface notes that the information contained in this guide
may differ from vaccine manufacturers' inserts, so when in doubt,
check the product insert. A product insert is a detailed description of
a pharmaceutical product and is included in each package of vaccine. For example, the section under "Fever" states that it is okay to
vaccinate a child with a "low-grade fever with or without mild
illness" but to wait if a child has a "fever with moderate-to-severe
illness" for any of the childhood vaccines. However, the product
insert from Merck & Co., sole manufacturer of MMR in the U.S.,
states that "any febrile respiratory illness or other active febrile
infection" is a contraindication for this vaccine. From other material
I've read, most doctors are cautious and will not vaccinate a child
with a fever, no matter how slight. It is precisely because of this that
the CDC recommends vaccinating children with low-grade fevers.
Why? To increase vaccination rates and opportunities for vaccination: a mother who has to come back later to get her child a shot is
less likely to return.
    So, while this booklet makes determining valid contraindica-
tions quick and easy, it tends to broaden the "yes" categories and

narrow the "no" categories that doctors may have been using in the past. As another example, a seizure within three days after receiving a DTP shot is not considered a contraindication but only a precaution against receiving future DTP shots. Similarly, an "underlying neurological disorder" (e.g., seizure disorders, cerebral palsy, and developmental delays) is also not considered a contraindication but only a precaution against receiving a DTP shot. (Read *A Shot in the Dark,* reviewed in Section B.2, for details on this). The doctor and parent are told to weigh the benefits and risks and make their decision. Parents must be aware of contraindications that would put their child at high-risk for adverse reactions so they do not receive a particular vaccine. However, how much medical history does a two-month old baby have? Or even a 15 month-old (the age the first MMR is given)?

This booklet is a good as a quick reference, but get copies of the product inserts from your doctor, as well, and take them home to read before your child receives a shot.

Available From:
National Immunization Program (1). Free.

The Hazards of Immunization
Sir Graham S. Wilson, M.D. London: Athlone Press. 1967. 324 pp.
ISBN 0-485-26319-X. Index. Bibliography.

Dr. Wilson was the former director of the Public Health Laboratory Service of England and Wales. He was a strong supporter of vaccination. However, he believed that unless doctors are aware of why vaccines failed in the past, similar mistakes may be repeated. In this book, Dr. Wilson lists all the vaccine failures that he accumulated over many years of correspondence with colleagues.

He organizes the book by cause of failure. There are chapters on faulty production, faulty administration, allergic reactions, and abnormal sensitivity of the patient, among others. Most of the causes of vaccine mishaps in the past have been due to faulty production from inherent toxicity, the presence of foreign toxins, or wrong cultures used.

Dr. Wilson realized that his work would be used by the "anti-vaccinationists" (it has), but he believed that that is a risk he must take; since, in all medicine human error can occur, awareness will prevent future mishaps. He strongly believed that all immunization programs should be subjected to constant scrutiny so that unnecessary practices would not continue.

This book is now out of print, but it is the only book I've found which details the history of vaccine failures.

Available From:
Out of print. Check a medical library or interlibrary loan.

Immunization, Benefit Versus Risk Factors
Developments in Biological Standardization Series Vol. 43
Edited by the International Association of Biological Standardization.
Basel, Switzerland: S. Karger AG. 1979. 475 pp. ISBN 3-8055-2816-7.
Index. Endnotes. Bibliography.

This book contains the report of the 36th symposium organized by the International Association of Biological Standardization (IABS) held in Belgium in 1978.

There are sections on each of the current childhood vaccines available for use in 1978 as well as other vaccines normally used only in developing countries. Several papers are presented in each section. The history of each disease is explained followed by evidence showing how effective the vaccine has been in reducing the occurrence of that disease.

Separate papers discuss concerns with adverse reactions. For example, one paper presents evidence showing that a larger number of adverse reactions to tetanus toxoid vaccine occur from vaccines adsorbed with aluminum than those adsorbed with nothing. The reason why vaccines are adsorbed with another substance is to boost antibody response.

Another interesting point, rubella vaccine is given to small children so that they will not contract rubella and possibly infect a pregnant woman and cause birth defects in the unborn child. However, as noted in this book and in other more recent books reviewed elsewhere here, the incidence of rubella among pregnant women has not changed since the introduction of the rubella vaccine.

There is a whole section on economic cost/benefit analysis. (For example, President Clinton stated in 1993 that every $1 spent on vaccinations saves us $10 in medical costs down the road.) One chapter actually gives mathematical formulas for determining risks versus benefits of vaccines (!).

A chapter on legal aspects of vaccination is quite informative. The author, a scientist from West Germany, is opposed to mandatory vaccination except for diseases where the vaccine has few side effects, the disease is quite infectious and life-threatening, and means of educating the public to voluntarily accept vaccination have failed. Then the state, in the interest of the health of all its citizens, may have the right to impose compulsory laws. Since the state imposes these laws upon its citizens for their own good, the state must be willing to compensate those victims who unfortunately suffer reactions to the vaccines. West Germany made it law in 1961 that citizens may make claims against the state for any damages due to vaccination. Here in the U.S., prior to passage of the National Childhood Vaccine Injury Act of 1986, your only recourse was to sue the vaccine manufacturer. A daunting endeavor. Unfortunately, receiving monetary damages from the NCVIA has proven to be daunting as well.

This book is extremely pro-vaccination, but the scientists are not blind. They know that vaccines have risks; they just believe that the risks are worth it compared to the misery caused by the diseases. They advocate continued research into safer vaccines. They also stress the need for research into the possible long-term ill effects of vaccination.

Each paper is referenced and noted with scores of medical journal articles.

Available From:
Out of print.

Immunizations: The People Speak!
Questions, Comments, and Concerns about Vaccinations
Neil Z. Miller. Santa Fe, NM: New Atlantean Press. 1996. 78 pp.
ISBN 1-881217-16-7. Bibliography. Updated in 1998.

This book is a collection of questions and answers compiled from
several national radio and TV interviews granted by Mr. Miller
during the past several years. He has transcribed the questions he
received on open phone lines from parents and health professionals
and organized them according to topic (e.g., a particular vaccine,
legal issues, etc.).

   The book is enlightening to read for the variety of questions
asked and the experiences and comments presented by the questioners. As Mr. Miller notes in the preface, parents have many questions
on this topic and are eager to receive information other than the
"standard line" from health professionals.

   Mr. Miller does a fine job of answering questions, especially
ones from people who attack his views. He does, however, let his
strong contempt for the medical establishment show through at
times, for instance when he refers to members of the medical establishment (not the average doctor, though) as "henchmen" and
"cronies".

   When questioners ask for advice regarding whether they should
receive such and such vaccine, he is quick to state that he does not
recommend for or against any particular vaccine. He only wishes to
present evidence for parents to decide for themselves.

   Topics covered by the questions include: discussions of the
safety and need for each of the childhood vaccines, possible long-
term effects, AIDS, government immunization programs, and legal
exemptions. The best part about the book is that you realize you are
not alone in having questions about the safety and effectiveness of
vaccines. It is best read after you have familiarized yourself with the
basic arguments for and against vaccines.

   He quotes liberally from different medical studies and attaches a
bibliography for readers to follow-up with their own research.

Available From:
Nelson's Books (8). New Atlantean Press (8).

Immunizations: The Terrible Risks Your Children Face That Your Doctor Won't Reveal

Robert Mendelsohn, M.D., GA: Second Opinion. 1994.
ISBN 0-96266469-3. Index.
Original title: *But Doctor, About that Shot...The Risks of Immunizations and How to Avoid Them.*

The late Dr. Mendelsohn, a pediatrician for 30 years, was an outspoken critic of modern medicine. He was also an outspoken critic of vaccinations. He edited "The People's Doctor" newsletter for many years and he prepared 12 newsletters on the topic of vaccinations. They were originally published from 1976 to 1988. They are collected together in this book.

Dr. Mendelsohn discusses adverse reactions to vaccines and their ineffectiveness. Most of his space is used answering questions from concerned parents, which I found quite interesting. Because this is a series of newsletters, the book is not cohesive and information on any one vaccine will be found scattered throughout (use the index). Much food for thought. Individual articles are amply referenced with medical sources.

Available From:
Out of print.

The National Health Federation's "Immunization Kit"

Fall 1994. This is a folder of vaccination article reprints and two books: *Vaccines: Are They Really Safe and Effective?* by Neil Miller and *Vaccination: Examining the Record* by Judith DeCava both reviewed in Section A.1. Prior to this folder, the "Kit" consisted of a spiral bound book of article reprints only.

This "Kit" has been revamped and now includes two books along with article reprints. Among the items included are: (1) an article by Tom Finn, Esq. on legal exemptions from receiving vaccinations; (2) an article by Richard Moskowitz, M.D. on how vaccines work; (3) the opening statement from the Senate hearing on the Gulf War Syndrome on the use of experimental vaccines on soldiers (this is very interesting and frightening); and (4) an article by Richard Leviton on political and legal issues.

Available From:
National Health Federation (2).

Vaccination Dangers
Compiled by Josephine Szczesny. Northbrook, IL: Vaccine Research.
200 - 300 pp. 8 1/2" x 11" binder.

Josephine Szczesny is the director of Vaccine Research, which
distributes information on the dangers of vaccination. This binder is
a compilation of newspaper and magazine articles, letters, and other
reprints about adverse reactions associated with vaccinations.

She includes copies of letters she has written to Congress
opposing mandatory vaccination laws and editorials criticizing the
vaccine political machine. There's a copy of a lengthy portion of a
government report titled *A Review of Selected Federal Vaccine and
Immunization Policies* (1979). Vaccine risks, adverse effects, and
vaccine injury compensation are covered.

She has a section containing resources for further information.
Ms. Szczesny does not systematically treat each vaccine. It is best
used as a reference for those who want to get a glimpse into the
political machinery and read more about adverse reactions. She is
continually adding new material to the binder.

Available From:
Vaccine Research (1).

Vaccinations: Deception & Tragedy
Michael Dye. Shelby, NC: Hallelujah Acres Publishing. 1999. 126 pp.
ISBN 0-929619-07-2.

This book is an attempt to tell the "truth" about vaccines and expose
the medical community's "cover-up" of vaccine failure. It does not
say in the book who Mr. Dye is, but at one point, it mentions that he
is with Hallelujah Acres. Hallelujah Acres is a Christian health ministry founded by Rev. George Malkmus. Rev. Malkmus advocates a
raw fruit and vegetable diet as stated in Genesis 1:29. (See their
website hacres.com for details on their diet). I assume, Mr. Dye is
also a member of this Christian ministry.

The purpose of this book is to tell readers about the adverse effects of vaccines. Mr. Dye believes this is necessary to counteract the almost 100% pro-vaccine material that inundates our society. He encourages readers to check his references and see for themselves that what he writes is true. Mr. Dye writes about the same topics covered in other vaccine books reviewed in this section, however, he rarely goes to the original source material for his information, instead he quotes heavily from other consumer vaccination books.

He asks whether vaccines are safe and details the possible connection between DPT and SIDS, the SV-40 contamination of polio vaccine, the 1976 swine flu mess, among others. He quotes heavily from Harris Coulter's book, *Vaccination, Social Violence, and Criminality* (reviewed in Section B.2), Viera Scheibner's book, *Vaccination* (reviewed in Section B.2), and Neil Miller's book, *Vaccines: Are They Really Safe and Effective?* (reviewed in Section A.1), and the NVIC website.

He asks if vaccines have helped reduce disease occurrence and presents data showing that diseases were already on the decline prior to vaccine introduction. Here he quotes from Dr. Mendelsohn's book, *How to Raise a Healthy Child. . .in Spite of Your Doctor* (reviewed in Section A.3), Leon Chaitow's book, *Vaccination and Immunization* (reviewed in Section B.3), as well as the books I listed previously. He covers legal exemptions to vaccination and quotes from Grace Girdwain's book, *Your Personal Guide to Immunization Exemptions* (reviewed in Section F). Another chapter details the possible link between vaccines, encephalitis, learning disorders, and sociopathic behavior. It is basically a summary of Harris Coulter's book, *Vaccination, Social Violence, and Criminality*.

He includes a very short two-page chapter explaining how vaccines are made. This is the weakest part of the book. It is vague and inaccurate. He states that "diphtheria vaccine" is collected from serum taken from a horse. This is how diphtheria antitoxin is made which confers only passive immunity. It was used in the early part of this century prior to the development of the diphtheria toxoid currently used in the DTP shot. While diphtheria antitoxin may still be available, it is rarely used today.

Mr. Dye shines, however, in his chapter detailing how our immune system works. Here he does a wonderful job explaining

how things work on a cellular level. He emphasizes how compli-
cated our immune system is and yet ordered and efficient. It is a
great gift from God so we can heal ourselves. My. Dye presents
evidence to support the idea that the state of our body's health is the
most important factor in its ability to fight off infections. He emphasizes the need for a proper diet, ala Hallelujah Acres, to provide the
body with the proper nutrients it needs to stay strong and healthy.
Mr. Dye, and Mr. Malkmus in the foreword, emphasize treating our
bodies with care, as God intended. This means following Natural
Law (God's laws written in nature) and following His word in the
Bible.

If you wish to read a summary of what other authors critical of
vaccines have written on this subject, Mr. Dye presents their conclusions here. He cites from each book or article in the text, but does
not include any references or a bibliography. Some of his cites are a
little vague, e.g., "a 1997 issue of such & such journal". Without a
bibliography, the reader is hard pressed to follow-up his references.
However, if his book encourages you to read more, then the authors
he quotes from are a good choice to start with. Overall, an interesting summary of the major arguments against immunizations and a
great explanation of our God-given immune system.

Available From:
Hallelujah Acres (2).

What Price Vaccinations?
Simone Delarue. English translation by Beate Boelter. Magalia, CA:
Happiness Press. 1992. 127 pp. ISBN 0-916508-22-6. Index. Originally
published in France under the title "La Rancon des Vaccinations".

The author, Simone Delarue, at the time of writing this book, was
the president of the French organization "League for the Liberty of
Vaccinations", which opposes mandatory vaccination laws. Although the copyright date is 1992, it has only been made available
in an English translation since 1996.

Ms. Delarue presents evidence bearing on the possible long-
term and short-term adverse effects of vaccinations. Much of her
material covers the use of the smallpox vaccine, which was

discontinued in the late 1970's after official worldwide eradication of smallpox. She explains her continued reference to the smallpox vaccine because it was the longest vaccine in use and, therefore has accumulated a long history of adverse effects. Also, she believes it is relevant because *vaccinia* virus is being considered for use as a "vector" (a sort of "host cell") for attaching antigens from different viruses in the development of new genetically engineered vaccines. *Vaccinia* virus is the virus generally used to make the smallpox vaccine, but the term can also refer to the cowpox virus, which is very similar to smallpox and also infects humans. She is very cautious of genetically engineered vaccines. She is concerned with the potential long-term effects these vaccines may have on our immune systems in this and succeeding generations. (See Section D for more information on genetically engineered vaccines.)

Ms. Delarue believes that vaccines are possible culprits in triggering many illnesses and diseases that exist today in such large numbers. In this regard she echoes Harris Coulter in his book *Vaccination, Social Violence and Criminality* (reviewed in Section B.2).

She cites evidence linking SV40 (simian retrovirus) contaminated polio vaccine administered in the late 1950's and early 1960's with the aggressive smallpox campaigns in Africa of the early 1970's. She believes that the smallpox vaccine triggered the dormant SV40 to become AIDS . (See Section B.3 for more information on this theory.)

Ms. Delarue is most concerned with viral vaccines, as opposed to bacterial vaccines, as viruses are much more complex and capable of attaching themselves to host cell genes. She also adds a chapter on a SIDS and DPT connection.

Ms. Delarue's references are mainly from French medical journals. Overall, a thought provoking book.

Available From:
Grain & Salt Society (8).

Section B.2

The DPT Vaccine

The whole-cell, killed pertussis vaccine has amassed a long history of adverse reactions since its introduction in the 1930's. Pertussis, or whooping cough as it is also known, is a respiratory illness characterized by a "whooping" sound made when one tries to breath. It can be very serious or fatal in the very young and lead to neurological damage. It is milder in older children and adults who may not be able to tell it apart from a bad cold.

It was the 1982 expose on a Washington, DC, TV station titled, "DPT: Vaccine Roulette", which triggered strong parental concerns about DTP, the founding of the parents group "Dissatisfied Parents Together" (DPT, now called NVIC), and prompted the eventual 1986 enactment of the National Childhood Vaccine Injury Act. It also led to the writing of many of the following books.

The medical community acknowledges the problems with the whole-cell killed pertussis vaccine, although they maintain that severe reactions are rare. The FDA approved the use of acellular pertussis vaccine in December 1991, which is supposed to have fewer adverse effects. However, it was only allowed for use in the fourth and fifth doses of the standard five dose DPT series (referred to as DTaP). The FDA approved DTaP vaccine on July 31, 1996 for use in the primary three dose series. So now, you can completely avoid the use of the whole-cell killed pertussis vaccine. Development of this new, safer vaccine was a goal of the National Vaccine Information Center (NVIC).

The books that follow address the DPT vaccine made with whole-cell killed pertussis and the controversy surrounding it.

Adverse Effects of Pertussis and Rubella Vaccines
Christopher P. Howson, Cynthia J. Howe, and Harvey V. Fineberg, eds.
Institute of Medicine. Washington, DC: National Academy Press. 1991.
367 pp. ISBN 0-309-04499-5. Index. Endnotes. Bibliography.

How did this book come about? Section 312 of the National Childhood Vaccine Injury Act of 1986 (PL 99-660) called for a review of
all relevant literature pertaining to adverse effects of pertussis and
rubella vaccines. The Institute of Medicine (IOM) conducted the
review, and in November 1989 established the Committee to Review the Adverse Consequences of Pertussis and Rubella Vaccines.
There were eleven members on the committee. All, except one,
were from various university medical departments. The committee
had to conduct a workshop and public meeting on the issue and pre-
pare a report of their findings. This book is their report. They have
sifted through a wealth of data, from journal reports and case studies, to information presented by concerned parents and organizations such as the NVIC.

The committee members attempted to determine whether certain
illnesses could be causally related to pertussis or rubella vaccines.
Since pertussis vaccine is almost always given as one component of
the DPT vaccine, they refer to DPT throughout the report. Their
basic findings are as follows: (1) they found insufficient evidence to
indicate a causal relationship between the DPT vaccine and a variety
of neurological disorders, including learning disabilities and attention deficit disorder (ADD); (2) they found no evidence to indicate a
causal relation between SIDS and DPT; (3) the evidence is "consistent with a causal relation" between DPT and acute encephalopathy
and an "unusual shock-like state"; and (4) the evidence "indicates a
causal relation" between DPT and anaphylaxis (a severe allergic
reaction to an antigen in the vaccine). Regarding rubella vaccine,
they found evidence to be "consistent with a causal relation" to
chronic arthritis, especially juvenile rheumatoid arthritis, and a
"definite causal relation" to acute arthritis.

Chapters include one on the history of the pertussis and rubella
vaccines and one on the methodology the committee used to evaluate the evidence.

There is a whole chapter on SIDS and DPT. They examine a
number of studies that suggest a possible link between SIDS and

DPT, but discard them all as flawed in some respect. Their final conclusion is that they can not determine that SIDS occurs with any more frequency after a DPT shot or in any consistent pattern after a DPT shot. In fact, they bring up evidence to suggest that there are fewer SIDS deaths just after a DPT shot so, therefore, the DPT shot may help reduce the overall incidence of SIDS. Their reasoning? Their belief is that other factors (e.g., low socio-economic status, a present or prior illness, or malnutrition) are probably a greater influence on SIDS deaths. Many SIDS deaths are in poor, minority families who probably have not immunized their children. Since few SIDS deaths occur in wealthier, white families, and more of them have had their shots, they suggest that the DPT shot may protect them from SIDS(!). Incidentally, the authors state that so far no study has conclusively linked apnea (periods when the baby stops breathing) to a predilection towards SIDS. However, Viera Scheibner in her book *Vaccination: The Medical Assault on the Immune System*, reviewed later in this Section, presents evidence making this connection.

The authors admit that more studies need to be done on all aspects of adverse effects from vaccines. The evidence they examined was spotty and inconclusive. In particular, they stress the need for a better understanding of the biological mechanisms behind adverse effects associated with the pertussis and rubella vaccines and with the natural infections. Also, they fault many of the studies for not including follow-up data, which would help to determine any long-term effects.

There is a lot of statistical analysis in this book. The authors only consider statistical evidence and never mention individual patient cases. There are literally hundreds of reports, books, articles, and case studies cited in the bibliography — 74 pages long! Extremely conservative in admitting any causal relationships, but they agree more research needs to be done.

Available From:
National Academy Press (8).

Pertussis: Evaluation and Research on Acellular Pertussis Vaccines
Developments in Biological Standardization Vol. 73
IABS Eds. Basel, Switzerland: S. Karger. 1991. 378 pp.
ISBN 3-8055-5457-5. Footnotes.

This volume contains the proceedings of an international symposium held in Japan by the International Association of Biological
Standardization (IABS) and the National Institute of Health of Japan
in September 1990. Symposium participants were mainly from
Japan, the U.S., and Europe. As this symposium took place prior to
the introduction of the acellular pertussis vaccine in the U.S., part of
the purpose of the symposium was to examine the success of the
vaccine in Japan where it has been in use since 1981.

Papers were presented on various areas of concern about the
vaccine. This included studies on how well the vaccine works,
development of the acellular vaccine in Japan, details of how pertussis toxin works in the body, and papers on clinical trials of the
vaccine. Papers also were presented comparing the whole-cell and
acellular versions.

Since Japan is the first country to have developed and used the
acellular pertussis vaccine, it is fitting that the symposium was held
there. In the 1970's, people in Japan became concerned about
adverse reactions from the whole-cell pertussis component of the
DPT vaccine. In 1975, the pertussis vaccine was suspended after an
accident occurred in which children died after receiving the vaccine.
Shortly after this, pertussis vaccine was resumed, but only in children two years of age and older. Researchers in Japan scrambled to
produce a safer vaccine for use in infants, and the acellular vaccine
was developed and made ready for use starting in 1981.

Pertussis rates rose among infants in the years the vaccine was
given only to those two years of age and older. It has decreased
again since introduction of the acellular vaccine. Japanese researchers at the symposium noted a rise in adverse reactions after the third
and fourth doses of the new vaccine and were discussing a move to
lower the primary series to two doses with one booster later.

One paper presents a follow-up on a clinical trial in Sweden in
1986 using the Biken acellular pertussis vaccine during which three
children out of 1,385 study children died at two, four, and ten weeks

after the shot due to severe bacterial infections from Hib, pneumonia, and meningococcal infections. The Japanese use the Biken vaccine as well, and in over six million injections to more than 1.5 million children, only one death has been reported. They state that they do not know why the children died in the Swedish trial and can not determine if the vaccine was related to the children's deaths. Participants at the symposium commented that Japan is more aggressive at treating bacterial infections with antibiotics than Sweden is and that that could play a part in the different results of use of this vaccine.

U.S. researchers at the time of this symposium were concerned about whether the acellular vaccine worked as well as the whole-cell killed one and whether it was safe. The Japanese were working hard to assure the scientists that this vaccine was a great improvement over the old, whole-cell vaccine.

This book is footnoted with scholarly works. Most papers were presented by those who did the research for that paper. This report is of interest to those who would like detailed information about the development of the acellular pertussis vaccine.

Available From:
Out of print.

A Shot in the Dark
Harris L. Coulter and Barbara Loe Fisher. NY: Avery Publishing. 1991. 246 pp. ISBN 0-89529-463-X. Index. Bibliography.
(An earlier edition was published under the title, *DPT: A Shot in the Dark.*)

The original version of this book, published in the early 1980's, was responsible for bringing the dangers of the whole-cell, killed pertussis vaccine before the eyes of the public. Harris Coulter and Barbara Loe Fisher concentrate solely on the "P" in DPT, i.e., pertussis, also called whooping cough. Emotional case histories from parents of vaccine-damaged children are interspersed with chapters on the history of pertussis, the history of the whole-cell killed pertussis vaccine, and the politics behind vaccination campaigns. Mr. Coulter is a medical historian. Ms. Fisher is a co-founder of Dissatisfied Parents Together, now known as the National Vaccine Information

Center (NVIC), a non-profit group, which promotes the development of safer vaccines.

The pertussis bacterium is a very complex and changeable organism. It easily changes into pneumonia or bronchitis and can affect the brain and nervous system. The vaccine is volatile and can mutate easily, so every lot of vaccine must be tested. The authors stress the crudeness of the whole-cell killed vaccine. It has one of the highest rates of severe short-term and long-term reactions of any of the childhood vaccines in current use. Serious short-term reactions from DPT include high-pitched screaming, seizures, anaphylactic shock, and even death. Less obvious long-term reactions have also been attributed to the vaccine. These include learning disabilities, hyperactivity, autism, and allergies.

The authors stress the need for a safer vaccine and discuss the politics behind the delay in development of a safer one. They believe that vaccinations work, but that the whole-cell, killed pertussis vaccine is too crude to continue using. An acellular pertussis vaccine was approved in December 1991 for use in the 4th and 5th doses and on July 31, 1996, it was approved for use in the first three doses of DPT, as well. The acellular pertussis vaccine contains only the inactivated antigen, and not the other portions of the bacterium cell, which caused the bad reactions.

One of the main purposes of this book is to identify children who are at high-risk for severe reactions from a DPT shot and therefore should not receive this vaccine. The authors cover in detail the conflicting criteria which government agencies and drug companies allow as contraindications for receiving DPT. The authors believe that parents should be fully informed about contraindications to save their children from needless vaccine injuries and deaths.

The authors spend a whole chapter detailing the under-reporting of vaccine adverse reactions by doctors. The authors also discuss the way vaccine manufacturing is regulated by the government and the problems with the current system. The history of mandatory vaccination laws in the U.S. is covered as well.

The authors do not discredit the use of vaccines or the theory behind them. In fact, they state that in third world countries, the very real risk of death from pertussis outweighs the risks of the vaccine; however, in the western world this may not be so. The authors relate that in Sweden and West Germany, where the pertussis vaccine is no longer mandatory, incidences of pertussis have increased, but the cases have been mild with few or no deaths. Pertussis is a cyclic disease with a strong rise in cases occurring every three to four years. Health officials in these countries believe that even with increased occurrences, the disease here is safer than the vaccine.

This book is excellent. The case histories are real tearjerkers. Critics will argue that they are only "scare tactics", but you can skip the stories if you like. The book contains an extensive bibliography of medical journals, medical textbooks, and government documents, though, unfortunately it is not footnoted.

Available From:
American Vegan Society (2). Avery Publishing Co. (8). Center for Empirical Medicine (2). Homeopathic Educational Services (2). Koren Publications (8). The Minimum Price Homeopathic Books (8). NVIC (1). New Atlantean Press (8).

Vaccination, Social Violence, and Criminality: The Medical Assault on the American Brain
Harris L. Coulter. Berkeley, CA: North Atlantic Books and Washington, DC: Center for Empirical Medicine. 1990. 300 pp. ISBN 1-55643-084-1. Index. Bibliography. References.

Harris Coulter is the medical historian who co-authored *A Shot in the Dark* reviewed earlier in this Section. In this book, he presents the thesis that the vaccination programs started after WWII and continuing until today have caused our children irreparable brain damage. This damage ranges from lowered IQ, dyslexia, hyperactivity, learning disabilities, asthma, and allergies to severe brain damage, cerebral palsy, seizure disorders, sociopathy, and severe autism.

Mr. Coulter describes at length the various theories that have been postulated for the vast increase in these diseases in children since the 1940's. He believes that they all have a common cause: post-encephalitic syndrome. Mr. Coulter states that the most common cause of encephalitis in children today is from a reaction to the DPT shot, specifically the "P", or pertussis, component from the whole-cell killed version. This reaction may be as mild as a high fever after the shot or as severe as a sudden seizure. Mr. Coulter

believes that the lifetime effect of this little episode of, in most
cases, sub-clinical encephalitis is irreparable, neurological brain
damage. He estimates that 10% to 20% of the population may be
suffering from some type of mental and/or physical impairment due
to vaccinations.

Mr. Coulter backs up his claims with a generous use of footnotes. His sources are from medical journals. I would like to add
that this book is included in the bibliography for the IOM report
Adverse Effects of Pertussis and Rubella Vaccines, reviewed earlier
in this Section. It is also noted in the introduction to the IOM report
Adverse Events Associated with Childhood Vaccines (see review in
Section B.1). While no specific comments are made, it appears that
the IOM wishes to refute the conclusions that Mr. Coulter draws.

Available From:
Center for Empirical Medicine (2). Homeopathic Educational Services (2).
Koren Publications (8). The Minimum Price Homeopathic Books (8).
Natural Hygiene (2). New Atlantean Press (8). North Atlantic Books (8).

Vaccination: The Medical Assault on the Immune System
Viera Scheibner, Ph.D. Blackheath, NSW, Australia: V. Scheibner. 1993.
264 pp. ISBN 0-646-15124-X. Endnotes.

This book contains summaries of hundreds of medical journal articles regarding the effectiveness and safety of vaccinations. Dr.
Scheibner is a retired Principal Research Scientist in Australia with
a Ph.D. in Natural Sciences. In 1985 she and an electronics engineer
developed a breathing monitoring system for infants called
Cotwatch. It was from this project that she first became aware of a
link between the DPT vaccine, stressful breathing patterns, and
SIDS. Having no prior interest in vaccination, she undertook
researching countless medical journals to study vaccination for
herself. The result is this book.

Although the chapter on DPT is subtitled "A Cot Death Connection", Ms. Scheibner does not make this connection until the end of
this quite lengthy chapter. (Much of the contents are echoed in H.
Coulter's and B. Fisher's book *A Shot in the Dark*, reviewed in this
Section.) She includes a couple of graphs comparing several babies'

breathing patterns gathered from the Cotwatch system. I would like to have seen more data on more babies. Her findings regarding the Cotwatch breathing monitor are that a stressful situation, in this case a DPT shot, instigates a stress-induced breathing pattern that forms a predictable pattern over the course of several weeks. Some babies are unaffected by this stress, others have severe apnea (periods of non-breathing), and other babies' apnea is serious enough to result in a SIDS death. This pattern contains three elements: an initial alarmed reaction, a lengthy sustained reaction phase, and a final exhaustion phase where the child "gives up" and either dies or recovers from the stressful situation. This pattern is analogous to the body's general immune response to disease organisms. It is reflected here in the infant's breathing patterns. In a later chapter, she explains how the monitoring system was set up and worked. The implications of her findings are frightening if we consider the large number of SIDS deaths in this country. (The Institute of Medicine has not found a link between DPT and SIDS. See the review of *Adverse Effects of Pertussis and Rubella Vaccines* in this Section.)

In the rest of the book, Ms. Scheibner addresses each current childhood vaccine including hepatitis B and Hib, but not chicken-pox. There are also chapters on smallpox and flu vaccines. However, she doesn't discuss diphtheria and tetanus separately from the chapter on DPT (which is really only about the whole-cell, killed pertussis component of the vaccine). Ms. Scheibner summarizes medical journal articles that she believes show conclusively that there is little support for the belief that vaccines have anything to do with the decline in infectious diseases. She also lists many studies that indicate possible long-term effects such as atypical measles and cancers.

Ms. Scheibner's book is a slow read, since it is filled with a fair amount of technical medical terminology. All her research is from medical sources and everything is footnoted.

Available From:
Global Vaccine Awareness League (1). New Atlantean Press (8).

Whooping Cough, the DPT Vaccine and Reducing Vaccine Reactions
NVIC. VA: NVIC. 1989. 27 pp. Bibliography.

This booklet on the DPT vaccine was prepared by The National Vaccine Information Center (NVIC), a lobby group that supports research for a safer pertussis vaccine and other vaccines. However, the individual author(s) are not listed.

The authors indicate which children are considered "high risk", and therefore, should not receive the whole-cell, killed pertussis vaccine. They also list adverse reactions associated with the shot. They explain the National Childhood Vaccine Injury Act of 1986, which the NVIC actively sought for. This booklet condenses information from the book *A Shot in the Dark* (reviewed in this Section), minus the political information. It is not footnoted, but contains a bibliography of medical journal articles.

Available From:
Out of print.

Section B.3

Vaccination and the Immune System

The books reviewed in this section describe how vaccines affect the immune system. Some authors are afraid that vaccines weaken the immune system or harm it. Other authors implicate vaccines, for example, SV-40 contaminated polio vaccine in the early 1960's or the worldwide smallpox campaign of the early 1970's with triggering the AIDS epidemic.

The study of vaccines leads naturally to the study of the immune system and how our body prevents illness. I recommend that you read at least one general work on the immune system. We all would benefit from a better understanding of how our bodies fight disease. Our immune systems are amazingly complex; God's handiwork is truly awesome. I have to ask, are we not a little conceited to think that we can make our immune systems "work better" than God designed them by using vaccines? Are we foolish to try to "improve" something we barely understand?

The Case Against Immunizations
Richard Moskowitz, M.D. Alexandria, VA: National Center for Homeopathy. 1983. 22 pp. Bibliography. (Reprint of article from the "Journal of the American Institute of Homeopathy" 7 March 1983.)

Richard Moskowitz wrote this article to make public his arguments against mandatory vaccination. He has written other articles on the subject (see *Vaccinations: The Issue of Our Times*, reviewed in Section A.1). He is an M.D. who is also trained in homeopathy.

He states that since vaccinations are mandatory, there should be convincing proof that vaccines are safe and effective and that the diseases vaccinated against are serious enough to warrant these laws. He does not believe the evidence is there. Regarding effectiveness, he finds little evidence to support the claim that vaccines give life-long immunity, because too many people later get the disease that they have been vaccinated against. He concludes that immunity from a vaccine is only partial or temporary. (The medical community rationalizes that in some people a vaccine just doesn't "take".) He also lists several cases of vaccine-induced illnesses.

Dr. Moskowitz proposes that vaccinations may actually suppress the body's immune response as a whole. In the case of live virus vaccines, he suggests that the viruses may "hide" in body cells and appear at a later date as some other illness.

He also briefly covers the recommended childhood vaccines (except Hib, hepatitis B, and chickenpox). Many of his ideas are speculative, but he footnotes everything using mostly medical sources.

Available From:
National Center for Homeopathy (2). The Minimum Price Homeopathic Books (8).

Emerging Viruses: AIDS and Ebola, Nature, Accident or Intentional?
Leonard G. Horowitz, D.M.D., M.A., M.P.H. Rockport, MA: Tetrahedron, Inc. 1996, 1997, 1998. 594 pp. ISBN 0-92355012-7. References. Index.

This book attempts to answer the question of whether AIDS occurred naturally, or by accidental or intentional contamination of vaccines. Dr. Horowitz is a dentist, with a Ph.D. in dental science from Tufts University and a masters in behavioral science from Harvard. He previously wrote about AIDS in a book on the Kimberly Bergalis case in Florida called *Deadly Innocence*. This book is written as a first person account of his research. As an investigative reporter, he spent two years searching through medical journals, government reports, and interviewing individuals. He quotes extensively from his findings, which enables the reader to easily follow his investigation. Dr. Horowitz addresses both AIDS and Ebola, because they are similar diseases in that they both cause the immune system to fail. Ebola just does it immediately, while AIDS takes anywhere from months to years.

He is initially spurred on by the fact that in 1970, Congress released 10 million dollars for development of an immune system destroying biological weapon. He delves extensively into the circle of researchers who had access to and worked on cancer viruses during the 1970's. One of these was Dr. Robert Gallo, discoverer of HIV. Dr. Horowitz believes that cancer virus research in the early 1970's may have been tied into development of this biological weapon, or that the same researchers were possibly working on both things. Given the sudden emergence of AIDS in the late 1970's in both central Africa and New York City, he believes that it is highly plausible that the experimental hepatitis B vaccine may have been contaminated either accidentally or intentionally with HIV and given to homosexuals in New York City, while other vaccines used in Africa at the same time may have been similarly contaminated. Dr. Horowitz speculates that these populations were used as test victims for our biological warfare program. This theory is supported in the black community. (See Curtis Costs' book *Vaccines are Dangerous*, reviewed in this Section, for a view from the black community.) For critics who say that such an endeavor could not remain undiscovered, he supplies evidence suggesting that the CIA could easily have used just a handful of people to contaminate vaccine batches.

I think his evidence for an accident is stronger, as I tend to believe that most people spend their lives trying to do good, although some people's idea of "good" has at times caused great evil. For example, he includes congressional records from 1975 which expose CIA and military germ warfare experiments that took place from 1949 to 1969 on unsuspecting U.S. citizens through air tests of various bacterial and viral agents in cities around the country. Pretty horrible stuff. Even so, I am less inclined to believe conspiracy theories and more inclined to believe that human error, arrogance, or just plain messing around with stuff we don't really understand, could just as easily have led to the creation of AIDS or Ebola. Given that however, Dr. Horowitz raises questions that deserve to be answered.

I will focus on what he says about vaccine contamination as it has the most relevance for this Guide. Dr. Horowitz explains in detail how easy laboratory animals spread diseases among themselves and how animal tissue cell cultures can easily be contaminated with animal viruses. He presents documents with researchers discussing how difficult it is to keep cell cultures "clean". He explains the SV-40 contamination of polio vaccine in detail. This is the most thorough coverage I have seen of it. He gives details of how SV-40 was detected and excerpts from an interview of Dr. Maurice Hilleman, a top vaccine maker at Merck, discussing the SV-40 "problem". Although this incident is from the 1950's and early 1960's, viral contamination of animal cell cultures is still an ongoing problem in vaccine production. (The live and killed polio vaccines are cultured in monkey kidney tissues). His information echoes Eva Snead's book *Some Call It AIDS, I Call It Murder*, reviewed in this Section).

Regardless of whether or not you agree with Dr. Horowitz's speculations, the problem with contamination of cell cultures and vaccines is a real problem with unknown effects on our immune system. In the last chapter of the book, Dr. Horowitz talks about some of the scientists who are pointing at contaminated vaccines as possible instigators of autoimmune diseases, autism, and other diseases which have greatly increased in frequency in the last half of this century.

This is a wordy book, but it won't bore you. Dr. Horowitz meticulously documents all his sources. His material is from medical journals, government reports, conspiracy-theory books, interviews, and magazine articles, among other sources. Much of the book is speculative, but he presents the material so that the reader can ask questions too and come to his own conclusions.

Available From:
Healthy World Distributing (8). New Atlantean Press (8).

The Immune Trio

Harold E. Buttram, M.D., John Chriss Hoffman, Ph.D., and the staff of the Humanitarian Publishing Company. Richlandtown, PA: The Humanitarian Publishing Co. 1995. 5th ed. 192 pp. Footnotes. (Originally published as three separate booklets (hence the new title): *The Dangers of Immunization* by the staff of the Humanitarian Publishing Co., *Vaccinations and Immune Malfunction* by H.E. Buttram and J.C. Hoffman, and *How to Legally Avoid Immunizations of All Kinds* by Grace Girdwain.)

The Humanitarian Publishing Co. (previously, The Humanitarian Society and before that, The Randolph Society) was founded around 90 years ago to promote the natural laws of caring for the body and its mental, physical, and spiritual well-being. The Society, from its earliest days, has been opposed to vaccination. I wrote separate reviews of each of these three booklets in earlier editions of this Guide. I combine them together now.

Part I of the book was originally published under the title *The Dangers of Immunizations*. The authors argue against mandatory vaccination laws. The actual author(s) are not identified. However, it can be assumed that they represent the views of the Humanitarian Publishing Co. Drawing much evidence from Drs. Archie Kalokerinos and Glen Dettman of Australia, along with quotations from other medical sources, the authors present information that casts doubts on the safety of vaccines.

There's a brief chapter on how the immune system works and a chapter extolling the work of Antoine Bechamp and criticizing Louis Pasteur. Another chapter briefly describes each current childhood vaccine (except the new ones: Hib, hepatitis B, and chickenpox). A later chapter compares natural immunity with immunity derived from vaccines. The authors strongly support the theory that vaccines assault the body in ways very different from a naturally acquired virus or bacterium. The authors do not deny that vaccines work; however, they are concerned about the price we are paying in the form of a weakened immune system for the elimination of these childhood diseases. Their main argument is that since vaccines are not 100% safe and may possibly lead to future illnesses, they should not be mandatory. Individual quotations are referenced in the text so you can check their sources.

Part II of the book was originally published as *Vaccinations and Immune Malfunction*. The authors are Harold Buttram, M.D., a physician in family medicine and nutrition and John Chriss Hoffman who holds a Ph.D. in microbiology. The authors admit that much of what they are saying is hypothetical. They are merely putting forth their concerns in hopes that they will be studied further.

The authors are concerned that the immunity produced by a vaccine is inferior to natural immunity. They speculate that vaccines may "tie-up" many more antibodies than would be used if one acquired the disease naturally. This could cause the immune system to become weak and lead to susceptibility to other diseases down the road.

The authors also briefly discuss the problems with mandatory vaccinations and present ways to obtain legal exemptions. They propose a possible link between SV-40 contaminated polio vaccine, smallpox vaccine, and AIDS. One new chapter has been added to the original booklet. It is a very interesting chapter on the growing evidence in the medical literature of a link between live viral vaccines (OPV and MMR) and the rise of many new illnesses, mostly behavioral problems, which the authors believe could be related to the viruses bringing about genetic changes in our cells. They also are concerned about the contamination of these vaccines with the animal proteins from the animal tissues they are cultured in, and what effect these foreign proteins may play on our health.

The original booklet was footnoted, but the new edition incorporates the citations into the text. Sources used are medical journals, popular works, and alternative health books.

Part III of the book was originally titled *How To Legally Avoid Unwanted Immunizations of All Kinds*. It was prepared from a manuscript written by Grace Girdwain, although she is not listed as the author in the book. Ms. Girdwain offers valuable information on your legal right to refuse immunizations. She goes step by step through the process of obtaining a medical or religious exemption. No mention is made of philosophical exemptions, I assume because these are easier to obtain. She gives lots of advice for dealing with health and school officials. She stresses the crucial need to know the exact wording of your own state law and to follow that wording exactly in writing your exemption request. This is valuable information that all parents should be aware of.

Available From:
Philosophical Publishing Co. (previously The Humanitarian Publishing
Co.) (8). New Atlantean Press (8).

Immunity: Why Not Keep It?
Lisa Lovett, D.C. Australia. 1980's. 87 pp. Bibliography. (I received a
photocopy of this book from someone else, which unfortunately did not
contain the copyright page.)

Lisa Lovett is a chiropractor practicing in Australia. Her father is
also a chiropractor and never allowed his children to be vaccinated.
Dr. Lovett herself is strongly opposed to vaccinations.

Although the title of this book doesn't state it, one third of the
book is about vaccinations. Dr. Lovett starts with a chapter briefly
explaining how our natural defense system works and how vaccines
circumvent this system. She presents statistics, which many other
authors also present, showing that the incidence of infectious diseases was on the decline long before vaccinations were introduced.
She makes an interesting comment, that the very children most
likely to suffer a severe case of an infectious disease due to a weakened immune system through malnutrition, poor hygiene, or other
causes and who would therefore most benefit from avoiding getting
an infectious disease are also the most likely to suffer adverse reactions from the vaccine, precisely because of their weakened
condition.

In one chapter, she describes the common childhood vaccines,
but mainly explains how they may harm the immune system in the
long term. There are also chapters on the overuse and misuse of
antibiotics, AIDS, the benefits of chiropractic care, and the role of
nutrition in keeping your immune system healthy.

I noted one major factual error in the book. She describes the
pertussis vaccine as "a whole vaccine, which means the organism is
live". This is incorrect. Pertussis vaccine is a whole-cell KILLED
vaccine. In fact, the brief paragraph that this sentence comes from,
in which she describes what several different vaccines contain, is
not completely accurate in describing the other vaccines either.
Since I am familiar with this topic, I see these errors plainly. However, this alerts me, and it should the reader too, that there may be

other errors in the book dealing with topics I am less familiar with, and therefore can not pick out.

The book is footnoted and sources are from popular vaccination books and medical journals.

Available From:
Out-of-Print. She has completed a second edition, but it is not published yet. Contact Lisa Lovett (8) for more information.

Natural Alternatives to Vaccination
Zoltan Rona, MD. Vancouver, Canada: Alive Books. 2000. 64 pp. Resources.

This volume is part of the Alive Books Natural Health Guides series. Dr. Rona practices in Toronto, Canada, emphasizing preventative medicine and natural health. Dr. Rona is opposed to immunizations and in this book he offers his recommendations for natural ways to boost our immune defenses.

In the first half of the book, Dr. Rona explains why he disagrees with the use of immunizations. He states that there is little research on the long-term effects of immunization on our immune systems. He is concerned that vaccines may suppress the immune system and contribute to other childhood illnesses, like ear infections, allergies, or asthma.

He makes an interesting observation in his discussion on vaccines and autoimmune diseases. It is believed that autoimmune diseases occur when our body responds to a foreign invader that is similar to our own body tissues and our antibodies gets confused and start attacking our own body tissues. "Foreign invaders" are bacteria and viruses, which are all covered with a protein coat that our body does not recognize. However, it is theorized that sometimes small sections of a foreign protein (called an antigen) may be of the same structure as protein structures in our bodies (e.g., joints, cartilage,) and the body may produce antibodies to the foreign protein, but mistakenly direct these antibodies against our own tissues. What does this have to do with vaccines? Vaccines are made up of viral and bacterial antigens (the protein covering) sometimes whole or in pieces. It is these proteins that trigger the antibody response to the vaccine. Dr. Rona is concerned that the proteins in vaccines injected into the bloodstream may be a trigger for autoimmune diseases in children.

He describes the current surge in the number of parents refusing to have their children immunized. He believes that this is a natural reaction against a procedure that has unknown long-term safety and many known side effects. He also describes vaccine ingredients and their toxic qualities. His focus is on the immune system, and he summarizes current concerns in this area. He does not cover individual vaccines.

He describes what he believes are the best alternatives to vaccinations: proper foods and supplements to boost the immune system. He strongly supports breastfeeding. He encourages the use of organic foods and the good fats: omega 3's and 6's. He recommends avoiding dairy, processed and antibiotic-laden meats, and pesticide-covered foods. He recommends probiotic containing foods (e.g., yogurt) and some herbs as well, for example Echinacea. The second half of the book contains recipes emphasizing immune boosting foods.

I've never mentioned the physical aesthetics of any book I've reviewed before. But this book warrants an exception. All of its pages are glossy and most contain full-color photographs. All of the recipes are accompanied by beautiful, full-page, color photos of the dish. The book is stunningly published, a novelty among the books I review here, which without exception are all text and no photos.

The book is not footnoted. This is not a scholarly work, but Dr. Rona does list vaccine organizations, especially groups in Canada, that can provide more detailed information. It's a short book, but it is a good summary of current concerns about possible vaccine damage to our immune system with helpful recommendations and recipes for protecting our children's immune systems naturally without the use of vaccines.

Available From:
Alive Books (8).

The Role of Vaccinations in Immune Suppression, Cancer and AIDS
Teddy H. Spence, DDS, ND, Ph.D., D.Sc. Exmore, VA: Truth Seekers Press. 1995. 69 pp. No ISBN. Bibliography.

This book is actually a thesis project for one of Dr. Spence's degrees in nutrition. He decided to have it published in book form. The purpose of his thesis, as he states in the preface, was to compare the health status of vaccinated people with unvaccinated people. The results of this research are contained in the last twelve pages.

In the first few chapters, Dr. Spence presents quotes and statistics that support his view that vaccines don't work and that disease incidence was already in decline prior to the use of immunizations. He briefly covers the history of vaccination. He explains how vaccines affect the immune system and how this may be linked to AIDS, cancer, immune suppression, and neurological problems. Most of his sources are from other general vaccination books many reviewed here. For example, books by Cynthia Cournoyer (Section A.1), Walene James (Section C), Eleanor McBean (Section C), Eva Lee Snead (Section B.3), and Harris Coulter (Section B.2). This surprised me, since this was a thesis project.

The most important part of the book is his research project comparing the health of vaccinated and unvaccinated people. He sent out two questionnaires to unvaccinated people. The first one contained questions about general medical history, childhood diseases, eating habits, and environmental factors that might affect health. The second questionnaire, called a Biological Immunity Analysis, contained questions about the health status of various bodily organs and systems, and about vitamin and mineral deficiencies. Questions were also included on eating habits and type of water consumed.

He admits difficulty in locating unvaccinated people to partake in the study, particularly as some people are reluctant to let their non-vaccination status be known. He used statistics about the general vaccinated population as a control group. He does not say how many questionnaires were completed, but indicates that it was a very small amount. He lists the results of each of the two questionnaires in separate tables. Although he says copies of the questionnaires are included in the appendix, there is no appendix and thus no questionnaires, which makes it difficult to understand the tables. The findings suggest that the more vaccines a person has had the more illnesses and other health problems they have. He does mention too, that proper diet is an important factor in one's overall health, regardless of whether one is vaccinated or not.

Other authors critical of vaccinations have maintained that vaccinations may lead to an overall weakening of the immune system, resulting in more illnesses from other diseases; however, none that I know of have actually tried to prove this by conducting research such as Dr. Spence has done. I wish he had explained his project in more detail and provided more information, for example, how many took part in the study, and how he calculated his statistics. This is a fascinating preliminary study. Follow-up and monitoring of these unvaccinated peoples' health would be valuable.

Available From:
Truth Seekers Press (8).

Some Call It "AIDS" – I Call It Murder: The Connection Between Cancer, AIDS, Immunizations, and Genocide
Eva Lee Snead, M.D. San Antonio, TX: AUM Publications. 1992. Vol. I and Vol. II. 1000 pp. No ISBN. Footnotes. Index. Bibliography.

This is a detailed, lengthy book arguing that AIDS is a result of contaminated polio vaccine. Dr. Eva Snead is an Argentinean native who practiced medicine in the U.S. from 1965 to 1986, specializing in nutrition and holistic medicine. She started research on this book in 1986 after her medical license was revoked. Dr. Snead has searched through numerous medical journals, newspaper reports, and government documents obtained through the Freedom of Information Act. She wrote this book for the lay reader so she takes the time to explain medical jargon and procedures in lay terms.

Although this book is her explanation of how the AIDS epidemic started, it is so closely tied into worldwide vaccination programs that it belongs in this Guide. In the first part of Volume I, she explains that polio vaccine grown in green monkey kidney tissue was found to be contaminated with SV-40 virus picked up from the kidney tissues. This was discovered in 1960. Many of the millions of doses of polio vaccine administered before that time all over the world, presumably contained varying amounts of SV-40 virus. After 1961, the kidney tissue cultures were screened for SV-40 viral contamination and this is no longer a problem. Since then, medical researchers, who consider it an animal tumor virus because it causes cancer in laboratory animals, have extensively studied SV-40. It is theorized that SV-40 acts as a "helper virus" for other viruses making it easier for them to infect cells and, when combined with another virus, cause cancer.

After this section, Ms. Snead presents an overview of the history of AIDS and how it was discovered. She believes the official explanation to be a lie, since she is convinced that AIDS is "triggered" by the SV-40 contaminated vaccines. She shows only contempt for the medical establishment throughout the book.

The second half of volume I is devoted to vaccination. Dr. Snead discusses viral vaccines only, primarily the polio and small-pox vaccines. She quotes extensively from a 1967 meeting of the National Cancer Institute on the safety of using primary cultures versus cell lines in culturing live viral vaccines. Primary cultures are live cells taken directly from an animal. In the case of the polio vaccine, it is tissue from the green monkey kidney and in the case of the MMR vaccine, it is chick embryo tissue. Cell lines are cells grown in labs. These include human diploid cells. A diploid cell is a cell with the correct number of chromosomes for that species, i.e., a normal cell. The chickenpox vaccine is cultured in human diploid cells.

Dr. Snead exposes the problems with the unknown and unde-tectable contamination of primary cultures with viruses. She focuses on the SV-40 virus but also includes a long list of viruses known to infect chick embryos and calf serum (also used for some vaccines). What is most frightening is that she states that the laboratory people knew about these viral contaminants, yet reassured everyone that they could screen their cultures and make sure no contaminated cultures were used in vaccine production, although, as Dr. Snead contends, the tests used at the time for this purpose had already allowed viruses to pass by unnoticed. This is the most thorough examination that I have read of the possible problem with viral contamination of live viral vaccines. (Other books have addressed

SV-40, but not in detail and not mentioned any of the other possible viral contaminates.)

Volume II contains a lot of repetition from Volume I. In an early chapter, Dr. Snead details the attempt to create a live viral vaccine for adenovirus. Adenoviruses cause upper respiratory tract infections, though not as common as colds caused by other viruses. Experiments were done on military personnel in the mid 1960's with adenovirus vaccine grown in human embryo cell lines. The vaccine was discontinued after it was shown to possibly cause cancer. It combined with SV-40 already present in the body from contaminated polio vaccines received earlier, Dr. Snead contends. Dr. Snead also examines a link between SV-40 and leukemia. She believes that viruses (RNA tumor viruses) cause most cancers and she explains this in detail. (Just to present the "other side" of the SV-40 issue, Dr. Stanley Plotkin in his book, *Vaccines* (reviewed in Section E), discusses studies done on the SV-40 virus that do not show increased cancer risks among those individuals infected with the virus.)

She also includes a chapter alleging the use of vaccines as tools in chemical-biological warfare and another chapter relating the dangers of genetic engineering techniques.

This book is footnoted; however, the references in some instances are incomplete (which she apologizes for and explains) and the one for the 1967 NCI meeting that she quotes from at length, I can't even find. The book is very repetitious, containing repeated explanations and stories. The organization of the chapters appears haphazard. I truly think that this book would benefit greatly from a complete reorganization and serious editing to tighten the material, reducing the length by half (to a more manageable one volume), thus cutting the price of the book in half as well. If this were done it would be much more appealing to prospective readers, who if they are like me, consider 1000 pages a little much to wade through. This book raises important questions and deserves a wide audience.

Available From:
AUM Publications (8).

Vaccination and Immunisation: Dangers, Delusions and Alternatives
Leon Chaitow. London: C.W. Daniel Co. 1996. Rev. ed. 178 pp.
ISBN 0-85207-191-4. Index. Bibliography.

This book explains the immune system response to vaccinations. Oddly enough, the book never states who Leon Chaitow is, but other sources I have read indicate that he is a naturopathic doctor. He writes from Britain.

Mr. Chaitow covers the history of immunizations, refuting Pasteur in favor of Antoine Bechamp, as other authors have done. He includes several chapters on how vaccines are supposed to work, but do not. He discusses short and long-term adverse reactions. He does not cover each childhood vaccine individually; instead, he explains the theory behind vaccination. Of particular interest is a chapter on possible long-term effects of vaccines. These include cancers, altered DNA, multiple sclerosis, arthritis, etc. He presents scientific papers that suggest such possibilities. Another chapter offers ways to enhance the body's immune function through alternative health care. This includes homeopathy, osteopathy, acupuncture, as well as nutrition.

This revised edition includes a chapter on possible theories of how AIDS may have come to be. He relates the SV-40 theory. He quotes from Eva Lee Snead (I review her book *Some Call It AIDS... I Call It Murder* earlier in this Section) though he does not mention her book. He also does not list her in the bibliography, which has stayed the same as the earlier 1987 edition of his book.

It is referenced throughout with medical sources. He also uses much material from consumer vaccination books and alternative health books, which are listed in the bibliography. The revised edition contains a much-needed index, as well.

Available From:
The Minimum Price Homeopathic Books (8). New Atlantean Press (8).

Vaccines are Dangerous: A Warning to the Black Community
Curtis Cost. Brooklyn, NY: A&B Books. 1991. 119 pp.
ISBN 1-881316-08-4. Bibliography. Resources.

This is the first book that I am aware of that addresses the question of vaccination from the African-American perspective. It is a call to action to the African-American community against western white medicine. Mr. Cost holds an MBA from Northwestern University and has lectured and written about AIDS.

Mr. Cost wrote an earlier book on AIDS where he first details a possible link between AIDS and vaccination. He believes that AIDS is a biological weapon created by the white western world to stem the population growth of Hispanic and African peoples. This alleged plot was carried out by contaminating smallpox vaccines given to Africans and Hispanics deliberately giving them AIDS. He believes that this occurred sometime in the early 1970's. (Leonard Horowitz in his book, E*merging Viruses*, also reviewed here, speculates that illicit human trials of immune-system destroying vaccines may have caused AIDS.)

In a series of brief chapters, Mr. Cost reiterates his distrust of vaccines, stating that they do not work, they destroy the immune system, and they cause many ill effects. After each chapter he lists books for further reading. He also includes a series of photos of vaccine-damaged children and reprints of some materials from the NVIC sandwiched into the middle of the book. There are also a few short chapters on natural health and the importance of breastfeeding in building a healthy immune system in your child.

Mr. Cost is very conscious of racism and he hopes to encourage the formation of groups of African-Americans who will take medicine and health care into their own hands rather than continue to swallow what the white doctors have been selling them. I agree that all people — whatever their race — need to inform themselves about health issues and take a more active role in the care of their health.

At the end of the book, Mr. Cost lists references for further information on AIDS, vaccination, and natural health. Most of the books that he lists as references after each chapter or at the end of the book, are popular works on vaccination or health. Many of these

books are no longer in print (try your library), but he provides ordering information for the ones that are.

Available From:
Out of print.

Vaccines, Vaccination and the Immune Response
Gordon Ada D. Sc. and Alistair Ramsay Ph.D. Philadelphia, PA:
Lippincott-Raven Publishers. 1997. ISBN 0-397-58761-9. 247 pp. Index.
Bibliography. References.

This book, written by two Australian immunologists, is directed to
other researchers involved in developing new vaccines, particularly
virologists, microbiologists, and molecular biologists. Dr. Gordon
Ada has been an immunologist at the John Curtin School in
Canberra, Australia since the late 1960's. Dr. Alistair Ramsay, also
an immunologist, joined the School in 1988. They wrote this book
because, oddly enough in the past, immunologists have not been
closely involved in vaccine production. Drs. Ada and Ramsay
rightly argue that vaccine developers need to increase their understanding of all components of the body's immune system if they are
to be able to effectively manipulate immune responses through vaccination. The book is highly technical reading, but not impossible if
you want to read it alongside a medical dictionary.

The book is divided into six sections. Section one gives a brief
history of immunization, as well as descriptions of vaccines in current development (that's around 300 vaccines as of 1995). Section
two describes the immune system, emphasizing features relevant to
vaccination. Section three discusses the immune response to infectious diseases. Section four describes manipulation of immune
responses. Section five details the many new approaches to vaccine
development, i.e., "new generation" vaccines. Section six, the
authors believe, are the new and exciting arenas for vaccine use:
treating tumors and cancers, controlling autoimmune diseases, and
contraceptive vaccines. Although they do not raise any ethical concerns over the practice of artificial birth control in and of itself, they
do warn that "fertility control", by vaccination or other methods, can
be misused by groups for ethnic, cultural, religious, or economic

reasons (some-thing the pro-life community is well aware of).

I wish there were a comparable book written for the lay reader that addresses the latest findings on how the immune system works in relation to vaccines. (The best alternative I can suggest is the relevant chapter in Catherine Diodati's book *Immunization: History, Ethics, Law, and Health* reviewed in Section C). Drs. Ada and Ramsay have done a great service for vaccine researchers who will benefit from this overview of the latest findings on immune responses. This book is extensively footnoted with medical journal studies.

Available From:
Out of print

Section B.4

MMR and Hepatitis B Vaccines

B oth MMR and hepatitis B vaccines have amassed reports from people claiming they have caused a multitude of long-term adverse reactions.

For MMR, one of these possible effects is autism. Several national autism groups are actively addressing a vaccine-induced cause for the disease. (See listing under Health Organizations in Resources). The book reviewed below *I Don't Want to Be Ty* examines the possible link between MMR, specifically the measles component, and development of autism.

The first recombinant DNA hepatitis B vaccine was licensed in 1986. In 1991, it became the first recombinant DNA vaccine to be recommended by the CDC as a universal childhood vaccine. Since then, mandatory hepatitis B vaccine laws have been aggressively pushed by the vaccine manufacturers and health officials.

With increased use of the vaccine, reports have come in from around the country of serious autoimmune and neurological reactions to the vaccine. These reports are not just from children, but from adults who have received the vaccine, as well. The NVIC published a special report in the Fall of 1998 summarizing the current concerns with this vaccine. It is reviewed below.

Hepatitis B Vaccine: The Untold Story
Barbara Loe Fisher, ed. NVIC. "The Vaccine Reaction: Special Report".
Sept. 1998. 16 pp.

This report explains in detail the concerns that parents around the U. S. have about the safety of the hepatitis B vaccine. Ms. Fisher presents evidence proving that hepatitis B in the U.S. is little threat as an infectious disease. She also cites vaccine manufacturers' statements showing that the vaccine was tested for safety in several hundred five and ten-year-old children who were only monitored for five days following vaccination. Ms. Fisher states that the vaccine was never tested for safety on infants prior to its licensure. Long-term follow-up studies on safety have not been conducted and it is not known for how long a time the vaccine is effective. Given all of this, it is understandable that parents, who have accepted all other childhood vaccines for their children, are balking at this one.

Ms. Fisher quotes from medical doctors, nurses, and medical researchers who have first-hand knowledge of serious adverse reactions to the vaccine in themselves and among co-workers. Autoimmune diseases and neurological problems such as, autism, chronic fatigue syndrome, diabetes, arthritis, MS, and others are possibly adverse reactions to the vaccine.

The special report explains the role the CDC has in providing grant money to states based on the number of citizens who are fully vaccinated. The report also discusses vaccine-tracking registries. Ms. Fisher is truly frustrated over the apparent lack of concern among medical authorities about the safety of this vaccine.

Available From:
Out of print.

I Don't Want to Be Ty: A True Story of Vaccine Injury
Robin Goffe. 1999. Salt Lake City, UT: Utah Vaccine Awareness Coalition. 123 pp. References.

This book, written in story form, describes the first five years in the life of the author's son, Ty, who has been diagnosed with autism. Robin Goffe and her husband live in Salt Lake City.

The book describes Ty's childhood and how he was able to crawl, then stopped crawling, was able to talk, then stopped talking, and how he had many infections, some life threatening. It also chronicles the growing realization of the parents as they came to grips with the problems their son displayed. They were fortunate to be near medical specialists who were able to diagnose and treat their son for autism.

What strikes the reader the most is that Robin and her husband did much of the medical detective work themselves, tracking down studies and information at a university medical library near them. It was through a careful recalling of Ty's medical history that they were able to point the finger at the various childhood vaccines Ty had received, as the cause of his problems. This realization is excellently brought out as the story unfolds. In particular, they believe that vaccines he received at 6 months of age weakened his immune system. He also has high antibody levels to measles, a characteristic of autism. He received an MMR at 14 months of age.

The Goffe's were fortunate to have had their son Ty picked to be in an autism study to test a new machine that performs an MEG scan, which can detect epileptiform activity. Epileptiform activity is seizures or electrical bursts in the brain that are undetectable as regular seizures. Until this test was performed, the Goffe's were unaware that their son was experiencing seizure activity.

This book puts a face on vaccine injury statistics. Ty is a real live person – not a number – with a family who loves him dearly. It is quite evident, that if his parents had not taken the initiative and gone to search for answers themselves, Ty may not be with us today.

The Goffe's have been able to help their son. His immune system is stronger and his autism symptoms have lessened. He is talking again. What remedy are they using? After trying one route and contemplating another, Mrs. Goffe stumbled upon – or rather, was led by God – to consider breast milk (!) Yes, she is receiving donations of breast milk from a group of dedicated local mothers. I find it amazing what breast milk can do. Ty was four when he started the breast milk.

The book is footnoted where Mrs. Goffe refers to specific medical studies from her research. This book deserves serious consideration from the medical community, especially regarding vaccine safety and alternative ways to treat autism. Its message is particularly effective and thought provoking because the book is in story form. Mrs. Goffe is not overly emotional. She just details her family's experiences in hopes that this information may help others.

Available From:
Utah Vaccine Awareness Coalition (1).

Section C

Philosophical Objections

Some people oppose vaccinations for philosophical reasons. By this I mean they disagree with the medical theories that immunizations are based upon. For these people concern over adverse reactions is secondary. Vaccination is seen as one aspect of the way conventional medicine views disease, with its emphasis on eradicating disease organisms, instead of strengthening the body and its defenses. This latter emphasis is advocated by natural healing philosophies.

Some of the authors of books reviewed in the previous two sections are proponents of alternative health philosophies, in particular, homeopathy, naturopathy, and Natural Hygiene. I include authors in this section who focus mainly on presenting theories of health and disease, instead of critiquing individual vaccines. They believe in treating the body-mind-spirit as a total unit. Rather than focusing on "disease states", they focus on "health states" and maintaining balance in the body. You may agree or disagree with their conclusions. You may want to read more about the healing philosophies that they promote. Whatever you think, you will quickly see that they approach disease from a fundamentally different viewpoint than does conventional medicine.

Other Theories of Disease

Many authors critical of vaccinations reject the germ theory of disease. The germ theory of disease is the "one germ – one disease" idea, i.e., a specific germ causes a specific disease. In other words, germs invade our bodies from outside and make us sick. Louis Pasteur, who lived and worked in 19th Century France, is considered the father of the germ theory.

Instead, most of these authors believe that germs live in balance within our bodies until some factor disturbs that balance and leads to the uncontrolled growth of unwelcome germs. (They tend to use the term "germs" without defining it, but I assume they mean both viruses and bacteria.) Dr. Antoine Bechamp, a contemporary of Louis Pasteur, presented this view: the state of the body, not the exposure to disease-causing germs, is what determines if one will "catch" a disease.

The body's efficiency at excreting waste matter, they believe, is the crucial factor in keeping a person's body healthy. Germs feed upon the waste material produced by our bodies. When too much waste accumulates due to poor diet, lack of exercise, stress, environmental pollutants, or other factors that upset the body's equilibrium, germs feed upon this excess waste. Depending upon where the waste is located and which germs feed upon it, a different disease will result (e.g., colon cancer from toxic waste in the colon). In light of this theory, vaccines play no role because they contain toxic matter and therefore contribute to the body's load of toxic waste.

You will quickly note that many of these books are older and out of print. Why do I include them? Well for one, they give a historical perspective on the early anti-vaccination movement and its main reasons for rejecting vaccines. Also, these books and authors are sometimes referenced in other books you may read and it helps if you know something about them. To make it easier for the reader, I divide this section into two parts: Part I contains the newer books and Part II contains the older, mostly out of print books.

PART I: Newer books still in print

AHIMSA Magazine: Special Vaccination Issue
April/June 1995. Vol. 36. No. 2. Malaga, NJ: The American Vegan Society. 32 pp.

I don't ordinarily include magazines in this Guide, but since the entire issue of this magazine is devoted to vaccinations, I decided to review it. AHIMSA is published by the American Vegan Society. Vegans are vegetarians who use no animal source food at all or clothing from animals. They are the most vegetarian of the vegetarians. (This includes no honey, dairy, wool, or silk). AHIMSA is the Sanskrit term for non-killing, non-injuring. It is defined in modern terms as "Dynamic Harmlessness".

This issue of AHIMSA contains reprints of articles on vaccination that appeared in earlier issues. There's a lengthy 1986 review of Hannah Allen's book *Don't Get Stuck* (see my review in Part II of this Section). There are some news items on vaccinations from 1967 and 1972 issues. One article titled "Vegans and Vaccination" addresses the topic from that perspective and several others also reflect the Vegan/AHIMSA philosophy. There's an informative article on foreign travel for the unvaccinated and another on obtaining legal exemptions.

Included are short reviews of a handful of immunization books (most of these books they sell), all reviewed here (e.g., books by Mendelsohn, Neustaedter, Miller, James, Coulter, Murphy, and Cournoyer). While many of the books reviewed in Sections A and B contain much more detailed information, this magazine is of interest for the vegan/AHIMSA perspective brought to the subject.

Available From:
American Vegan Society (2).

Immunization: History, Ethics, Law, and Health
Catherine J. M. Diodati, MA 1999. Windsor, Canada: Integral Aspects, Inc. 312 pp. ISBN 0-9685080-0-6. Index. Footnotes. Bibliography.

This book examines mass immunization in Canada and other developed countries from a bioethical perspective. Catherine Diodati completed a shorter version of the book for her master's thesis titled "Biomedical Ethics: The Ethical Implications of Mass Immunization". This title more properly reflects the emphasis in this book. She was encouraged and helped in her research by the doctors on her thesis committee, especially when trying to understand complex immunological material.

This book does what no other I am aware of does. It examines the policy of mass immunization in developed countries against the four accepted criteria bioethicists use to judge a health service. She argues this against the idea that immunizations should produce utilitarian benefits. Utilitarian is defined as the greatest benefit for the greatest number is that which receives the greatest value. Whether mass immunizations provide a utilitarian benefit is explored by examining the bioethical principles of non-maleficence, beneficence, respect for autonomy, and justice.

Before she undertakes this examination, she includes a section on natural immunity and artificial immunity. She does a wonderful job explaining the complex terminology of immunology in lay terms and showing how our immune system works on the cellular level, as understood in current research. She then explains how artificial immunity works through passive and active immunization. She presents information speculating that immunity from a vaccine is quite different from natural immunity, especially in two areas: (1) it is not permanent, and; (2) it "uses up" more of the immune system than would be used in a natural infection. Her evidence for (1) is well known, since booster shots are needed for most vaccines. However, for (2) this is up-in-the air. I don't know if there is any hard data to confirm this. Even so, since vaccines can "wear off", obviously they do not work in our bodies the same as a natural infection does, so this is enough of a concern.

Ms. Diodati thoroughly examines the practice of mass immunization in light of the four principles of bioethics, which she carefully defines in the introduction to each of the four chapters. First, she presents evidence to support her argument that mass immunizations violate the principle of non-maleficence. Non-maleficence refers to the oath "first do no harm". Ms. Diodati contends that because immunizations are injected into healthy people who may or may not ever come in contact with the disease naturally and they contain potentially harmful substances besides the antigens (e.g., thimerosal, formaldehyde, contaminating pathogens, etc.) this violates the principle of non-maleficence.

Next, Ms. Diodati looks at the principle of beneficence, which means that the health measure should provide actual benefits. To see if mass immunizations have provided actual benefits, Ms. Diodati looks at the records of disease instance and fatalities, before and after vaccines were introduced, for the following diseases: measles, mumps, polio, and hepatitis B. She presents statistical evidence from Canadian health reports that show that disease cases were on the decline prior to vaccine introduction, and while the vaccine may have further contributed to a disease's decline, it was not the sole cause. Also, as she shows with measles and mumps, the average age one contracts the disease has risen, and the older one is when these diseases are contracted, the more dangerous they are. She concludes that mass immunizations have not provided actual benefits.

Immunization and respect for autonomy is covered next. Ms. Diodati defines respect for autonomy as the right of competent individuals to make their own choices in health care treatments. This means giving patients enough information to make informed choices and allowing them to decide without undue interference. She concludes that current major immunization practices in Canada violate both the right to make an informed choice, because all risks of the vaccine are not revealed prior to vaccination, and the right to decide without undue pressure, because of mandatory immunization laws.

Regarding immunization and justice, Ms. Diodati argues for a national vaccine injury compensation program similar to one we have here in the U.S.

Ms. Diodati is careful to define her terms precisely and explain her position. I can not state, however, that Ms. Diodati approaches her subject from a neutral position: her daughter suffered a severe reaction to her second DPT shot fourteen years ago. Her daughter was not left with any permanent disability, but this incident caused Ms. Diodati to become interested in researching vaccines. This may explain her eagerness to accept evidence in some areas that is speculative in nature.

Hers is the first I know of to present a lengthy, detailed look at the bioethics of mass immunization. While she limits her comments primarily to discussion of immunization practices in Canada, they're applicable with little modification to the U.S. and other developed countries. She does not however, apply this argument to vaccines in the developing world. That would entail a complete study of its own. She raises many serious questions about the continued practice of universal childhood immunization and her concerns deserve to be addressed by the medical community. I would not categorize her book as the complete word on the subject, but as a very important first step. I hope that this book receives a wide audience and its conclusions are met with serious discussion.

Because this book is based upon a master's thesis it is a scholarly work, but not overly technical. Ms. Diodati is very careful to footnote all her material and even includes copious notes within her footnotes. She has done a lot of research. Her source material is drawn from Canadian and other government health documents, medical textbooks and journals, newspapers, and consumer books.

Available From:
Integral Aspects, Inc. (8). New Atlantean Press (8).

Immunization: The Reality Behind the Myth
Walene James. Westport, CT: Bergin & Garvey. 1995. Second edition. 285 pp. ISBN 0-89789-360-3. Index. Footnotes. Resources.

Walene James, a mother and freelance writer, presents a detailed explanation of philosophical objections to vaccination in this book. She explores different ways of looking at disease and makes a convincing argument for a holistic view of health and health care in which vaccination plays no part.

In Part I she describes the known and unknown, but suspected, short and long-term effects of vaccinations. She briefly explains how vaccines work in your body differently from a natural infection. She offers advice in treating the "vaccine preventable" childhood diseases with natural remedies, especially with large doses of Vitamin C.

In Part II she explains the germ theory of disease and presents the alternative theory of Antoine Bechamp. This is a good summary of these two differing views. New to the second edition is a whole chapter devoted to what she terms the "new biology". This is more recent research by scientists who support Antoine Bechamp's. She presents the work of the German doctor Guenther Enderlein and a Canadian biologist, Gaston Naessens. This is one of the most interesting and important chapters in the book and I know of no other authors reviewed here who address current research in this area.

Part III is particularly informative. Here Ms. James explains in detail the 1981 court battle that her daughter fought to exempt her 2-½ year old son from immunizations. Ms. James' daughter was finally able to keep her son from getting his shots by obtaining a medical exemption. Ms. James also discusses her unsuccessful attempt to have a philosophical exemption added to the law in Virginia. It was her defeat in this matter which led her to write the first edition of this book, so she could educate more people about the existence of alternative views of health and disease.

Ms. James also discusses the power of words and the use of propaganda to promote mass vaccination campaigns. She states that it is time that we wake up from the "authority mystique" surrounding the medical establishment and become aware of how the words used by them shape our view of vaccinations. Or example, it is said that vaccines "wipe out" disease, or those concerned about adverse reactions are told vaccines are a "healthy risk", etc.

In another chapter, Ms. James presents detailed advice for readers who want to change mandatory immunization laws in their state, specifically to either add, or keep from losing, the philosophical exemption clause. She explains how to start a support group and gives examples of information you might wish to use and how to contact the media and legislators.

This is an excellent summary of philosophical objections to vaccination. It is heavily footnoted. Her sources are mostly popular health books, newspapers, and medical journals. I will add though, that she does use a number of quotes from sources that were quoted in other general vaccination books, but she notes this in the footnote indicating to the reader that she did not actually read the original source. (See my discussion of this practice in the introduction to the book reviews). However, aside from that, this book is excellent reading for anyone who wants to get beyond considering only the safety and effectiveness of vaccines, and wants to examine alternative theories of health and also learn strategies for making changes in our mandatory immunization laws.

Available From:
American Vegan Society (2). Greenwood Publishing Group (8). The Minimum Price Homeopathic Books (8). New Atlantean Press (8).

Immunization Theory vs. Reality:
Expose on Vaccinations
Neil Z. Miller. Santa Fe, NM: New Atlantean Press. 1996. 157 pp.
ISBN 1-881217-12-4. Index. Bibliography. References. Updated: 1999.

Mr. Miller has written two other books on vaccinations besides this one (see reviews in Sections A.1 and B.1). This is not an "introduc tory book" on the subject as was his first book, *Vaccines: Are They Really Safe and Effective?* (see review in Section A.1). It is mostly an indictment against the medical establishment, which he believes purposefully uses various "ploys" to convince people to vaccinate even though the establishment knows, Mr. Miller contends, that vaccines don't work and can harm or kill children. Mr. Miller uses emotionally-charged words and excerpts from letters he has received from parents whose children have died after receiving vaccines or who are now vaccine-damaged. This makes the book very powerful in convincing people not to vaccinate their children, which is why his first book, which isn't so emotional, is better as a "first read".

In a long section titled "ploys", Mr. Miller gives examples of various strategies vaccine policy makers, the medical community, and the government use to deny that vaccines don't work, to cover-up statistics, and to convince people to get shots. He deplores the use of coercion. For example, he mentions what he calls the "surprise attack". This is when a child is seen by a doctor for what-ever reason (e.g., an emergency room visit) and the immunization status of the child is asked (and the immunization status of any other children who happened to tag along), and immunizations are practi-cally forced upon the child while the parent is usually not emotion-ally equipped to deal with the situation at the present moment. Mr. Miller presents the ugly side of this practice, which is part of the CDC's *Standards for Pediatric Immunization Practices* (reviewed in Section A.2) and is strongly promoted as a way to increase immu-nization rates. Pro-immunization materials promote this practice as a good way to catch "poor, ignorant" parents who have "neglected" to immunize their children.

Mr. Miller derides the vaccine manufacturers concerning the Hib vaccine, which initially was given to two-year-olds, when the CDC admitted that 75% of Hib cases occur before age two.

According to Dr. Stanley Plotkin in his book *Vaccines* (reviewed in Section E) the vaccine manufacturers were working very hard to create a vaccine which would be effective in younger children. Children under age two are unable to make antibodies to the Hib bacterium, whether caught naturally, or obtained in this first Hib vaccine. Finally, a new conjugated vaccine was created in 1988 that was effective in younger children. Mr. Miller, incorrectly, condemns this age changing as somehow indicating that the CDC "couldn't make up its mind" at which age to give the vaccine.

This book is of value to parents who are already opposed to immunizations and want to be aware of medical "ploys" by people who want to convince them to vaccinate their children. He effectively uses fear by including letter excerpts from parents of vaccine-damaged children, which is why I would not recommend reading this book until you have decided whether or not to vaccinate. The book is well footnoted and researched with medical sources.

Available From:
Global Vaccine Awareness League (1). Nelson's Books (8). New Atlantean Press (8).

Mass Immunisation: A Point in Question
Trevor Gunn. Ulverston, England: Cutting Edge Pubs. 1992. 32 pp. ISBN 0-9517657-1-X. Bibliography.

This booklet is a summary of the writings of other consumer books on immunizations, in particular Walene James' book, *Immunization: The Reality Behind the Myth* (reviewed earlier in this Section). Trevor Gunn is a graduate in medical biochemistry and a practicing homeopath. He resides in England.

He gives brief coverage of the germ theory of disease and problems with it. He examines the common childhood vaccines and cites statistics that the rates of diseases were already falling before vaccination started. He contends that vaccines are ineffective as large percentages of vaccinated children may catch the disease vaccinated against in an epidemic. He supports the need for proper nutrition, hygienic environment, and abstinence from toxins as the only ways to insure a healthy immune system.

This booklet is of use to parents who are looking for a brief introductory booklet before reading more detailed material.

Available From:
American Vegan Society (2).

The Sanctity of Human Blood: Vaccination i$ not Immunization
Tim O'Shea, DC. San Jose, CA: New West. 1999. 80 pp. ISBN 1-929487-00-2. Bibliography. (Nov. 2000 revised edition. 127 pp.)

This book is actually a chapter taken from the book *Alternative to Annihilation: Considerations for Human Survival to Y3K*. I have not read this larger work and no summary of it is included in the present book. Tim O'Shea is a chiropractor. I review the first edition, but the third edition is now available. Dr. O'Shea is opposed to vaccinations. His book appears to be directed at people who have never thought to question vaccinations before. He urges all readers to check his sources and to "follow the money". At the beginning of the book, Dr. O'Shea does a very good job of pointing out problems on both sides of this issue. He states that "both sides get very shrill, emotional, and unscientific" at times. He explores what he contends are the motives behind why vaccines are mandatory: money for the pharmaceutical companies.

Dr. O'Shea explains that because human blood feeds all our cells, to inject any type of poison directly into the bloodstream violates its sanctity. Hence the title of this book. Dr. O'Shea does not believe that vaccines provide immunity the same way as natural immunity. He makes an interesting point, also brought out by other authors in Section C in particular, that because the disease organisms in live vaccines are so weakened so as not to cause the body to have an acute inflammatory immune response, they do not "attack" the body in the same way as the wild virus would. This is unnatural, he states, and therefore permanent immunity can not be attained.

Most of his material is gathered from other non-technical, or consumer vaccination books, in particular, books by Harris Coulter, Walene James and Neil Miller (all reviewed in other sections in this Guide). The only extensive primary source material he uses is a Facts on File report of International Mortality Statistics from 1981.

He uses this report to illustrate that disease incidences were declining prior to the start of immunizations. I noted at least one error: when discussing the influenza vaccine he confuses it with the Hib vaccine. Anyone who is unfamiliar with the vaccination controversy and who reads this book will be challenged to read more to be able to either refute him or agree with him.

Available From:
Koren Publications (8). New West (8).

The True Story: Germs, Infections, Epidemics and Vaccinations
Dr. William Holub and Claudia Holub. NY: Vaccination Alternatives. 1980. 17 pp. Bibliography. 8 ½" x 11" stapled pages. Chapter excerpted from *Healing: AIDS, Sex and Germs*.

Dr. William Holub is a nutritionist with a doctorate in clinical biochemistry. He has written several books on health. In this excerpted chapter from his larger work *Healing: AIDS, Sex and Germs*, Dr. Holub attacks the germ theory and completely opposes vaccination.

Dr. Holub believes that we are born containing all the "germs" that exist in the world (we all have herpes virus, syphilis virus, etc.). Germs exist to consume dead tissues and convert them back to dust. (In this chapter, Dr. Holub does not specify whether he uses the term "germs" to mean only viruses, or viruses and bacteria). When our bodies are malnourished, or the body's balance is upset by some factor (e.g., air pollution, environmental toxins, weather changes, stress, etc.) the germs in our body "eat" the decaying and dead tissues that this imbalance causes. They are "cleaning house". When this happens we call it disease. Because he believes that all disease comes from within, vaccination becomes a ludicrous idea, since it is based upon protecting the body from an outside invader.

Dr. Holub believes that our time and money would be better spent on insuring that our bodies function at their peak potential by eating fresh foods, exercising, and cultivating spiritual relationships.

Unfortunately, nothing is footnoted or referenced, so you can not examine the sources for his ideas. There is, however, a bibliography of suggested reading material.

Available From:
Out of print.

Vaccination: The "Hidden" Facts
Ian Sinclair. Ryde, New South Wales, Australia: Ian Sinclair. 1993.
4th Edition. 110 pp. ISBN 0-646-08812-2. Bibliography.

This book is an import from Australia written in the same vein as
others who espouse the Natural Hygiene philosophy (e.g., Hannah
Allen, whose book *Don't Get Stuck* is reviewed in part II of this
Section). Ian Sinclair operates a Natural Healing School in New
South Wales. He has researched the vaccination issue for nine years,
ever since his son was vaccinated as a baby.

Mr. Sinclair laments the lack of information on vaccines available to Australian parents. He wrote this book to fill that void. Much
of his material is drawn from U.S. and British sources. Similar to
other introductory books on vaccination reviewed in Section A, he
describes each vaccine and summarily rejects them all as causing
adverse reactions or not working at all. He uses a profuse number of
quotations from medical journals and consumer vaccination books
to back his claims.

Mr. Sinclair's section about the germ theory and Natural
Hygiene is very informative. He repeats himself a lot, but does a
great job of explaining why he believes that the "one germ – one
disease" theory is insufficient.

Mr. Sinclair points out that statistics used to suggest that vaccines have been responsible for the drastic decline in the number of
people getting a disease do not tell the whole story. He states that
many pro-vaccine or medical texts show only the years from the
turn-of-the-century or from the 1940's onward and the rapid decline
evident after a vaccine was introduced, but they ignore the years
prior, which show that the incidence of all these infectious diseases
had been declining for the past century or longer. I examined the
graphs in pro-vaccination books and, yes, many only include figures
for recent years, supposedly, because figures for earlier years are
unavailable, inaccurate, or incomplete. Mr. Sinclair uses this information to make his point that better nutrition and sanitation are what
have stopped the spread of infectious disease not vaccines.

The bibliography contains mostly consumer health books and consumer vaccination books that he encourages readers to examine. He does not include in the bibliography all the sources (many from medical journals) which he quotes in the text.

Available From:
Ian Sinclair (8).

Part II: Older, mostly out of print books

Don't Get Stuck! The Case Against Vaccinations and Injections
Hannah Allen. Fl: Natural Hygiene Press. 1985. 2nd Ed. 238 pp.
ISBN 0-914532-33-2. Index. Bibliography.

The late Hannah Allen was president of the American Natural Hygiene Society (ANHS). In this book, she writes about the Natural Hygiene view of disease and its opposition to vaccination. Ms. Allen debunks the germ theory and describes how she believes the body's defense system works. She does not discuss individual childhood vaccines. According to ANHS president, James Lennon, her views on vaccines and the germ theory do not reflect current ANHS thinking which he summed up in a letter to me, as "we believe parents should have the right to decide whether to vaccinate their children". They are opposed to mandatory vaccinations, but have shifted away from criticism of the germ theory.

Ms. Allen has a detailed chapter on the history of vaccination and another one on the swine flu incident of 1976. She includes several chapters listing case histories of people who reacted to vaccines or got diseases prompted by a vaccine (many of these are included in McBean's *The Poisoned Needle*, reviewed in Part II of this Section). She describes the Natural Hygiene view of healthful living. She also has two chapters on obtaining legal exemptions from vaccinations and includes sample exemption letters.

Some bibliography entries are incomplete, (e.g., dates are missing) and most of her references are from consumer health books, consumer health magazines, and popular vaccination books.

Available From:
Out of print.

The Poisoned Needle
Eleanor McBean. Mokelumne Hill, CA: Health Research. 1957. 199 pp.
No ISBN. Index.

The late Eleanor McBean was a nurse and naturopathic practitioner.
She wrote several books on vaccination. She was a strong proponent
of Natural Hygiene.

Since this book was written in the 1950's, Ms. McBean concen-
trates on smallpox and polio vaccines. She cites case after case of
people dying from the disease the vaccine was meant to protect
against, or from some other disease (cancer, skin disease, etc.) all
prompted, she believes, by the vaccine. She has a long section on
the Salk killed-virus polio vaccine where she lists many cases of bad
reactions. This section has been reprinted as a separate booklet titled
The Hidden Dangers of Polio Vaccine. This vaccine may now be of
interest again. It was rarely used after development of the Sabin oral
polio vaccine, however, as of January 2000, the CDC recommends
that inactivated (killed) virus polio vaccine (IPV) be used by children for the primary doses. This is not the same Salk vaccine of the
1950's but a more powerful and effective version.

Ms. McBean is not only opposed to the germ theory, but even
goes so far as to state that viruses do not exist. According to her, it's
all a concocted story by the medical establishment.

She has a highly emotional writing style. She includes no footnotes or bibliography, but she does quote liberally from many
doctors who have written against vaccination during the first part of
this century, and who support her views. (Many of these doctors
wrote books opposing vaccination.) This shows that opposition to
vaccination is not new and has existed during all of this century and
before.

Available From:
Out of print.

Vaccination Condemned
Elben (Eleanor McBean). Los Angeles, CA: Better Life Research. 1981.
Book One. 500 pp. Index.

This book was written by Eleanor McBean under the pseudonym
'Elben", apparently to shield herself from attacks by medical
authorities. She researched vaccinations for 30 years and wrote
several other books and booklets on the topic through the years, but
this is her major – and final – work. A second volume was planned
and is outlined in this volume; unfortunately, Ms. McBean passed
away before it was completed. I reviewed two of her other books in
this Section and this book is similar in tone and content to those
other two, that is, highly alarmist, emotional language and most
information on vaccine mishaps and adverse reactions are drawn
from experiences with vaccines that are no longer in use.

Ms. McBean believes that the sole motive behind compulsory
vaccinations is money. She alleges that all "vaccine-preventable"
diseases have actually increased since vaccinations. (She is especially referring to smallpox here). Most other authors opposed to
vaccinations, however, agree that disease incidence has fallen since
vaccines were introduced, even though they might argue about the
reasons for this.

She only examines smallpox, diphtheria, tetanus, and measles
vaccines at length. The chapter on diphtheria vaccine I found rather
misleading. She follows diphtheria vaccine with the initials "DPT"
but doesn't discuss the "P", i.e., pertussis, component. (She discusses tetanus in a separate chapter). The diphtheria vaccine which
she states as being an utter failure is actually diphtheria antitoxin
which was used early in this century and gave only passive immunity of short duration. It is not and never was part of the DPT vaccine. Diphtheria toxoid, first developed in 1926, is prepared differently and is used in DPT. The antitoxin did cause significant allergic
reactions due to the horse serum it was drawn from. In another
chapter, she describes how diphtheria antitoxin is made and states
that this is the substance used in DPT. It is not. To give her credit,
however, her description of how polio vaccine is made appears to be
fairly accurate.

The same problem with the chapter on diphtheria vaccine
appears in the following chapter on tetanus vaccine. She charges

that the tetanus vaccine causes tetanus. All the cases she quotes to support this are from the 1920's or earlier. Until 1938, when tetanus toxoid was first made, only tetanus antitoxin was available. This conferred passive immunity of limited duration and was drawn from horses infected with tetanus. There were many instances of allergic reactions to the horse serum. Tetanus antitoxin is not used in DPT, only the toxoid, which is not made from horse serum. Ms. McBean either is unaware of this, or ignores this fact, as she presents her evidence from the 1920's and earlier to refute the use of tetanus vaccine for today. Her many case reports are of historical interest in illustrating the problems with vaccine manufacturing in the early part of this century when methods were crude and not well regulated.

She includes a lengthy chapter on measles vaccine, but in the second half of the chapter she does not distinguish between measles vaccine and German measles vaccine (rubella). She correctly states that the killed measles vaccine was linked with cases of atypical measles, but says it is still in use. However, after the report was published linking the killed measles vaccine to atypical measles cases in 1967, this vaccine was discontinued. By this time, tens of thousands of children had already been vaccinated in the years it was in use, 1963-1967.

Ms. McBean repeats many times that measles cases increased after vaccination. While it may be true that the danger of contracting measles was exaggerated to scare people into getting vaccinated, she presents her statistical data haphazardly. An orderly, well-documented presentation using graphs would make her case much stronger and this is true throughout the book.

She includes several chapters exposing the tactics of medical authorities whom she believes exaggerate the dangers of disease and create false epidemics in order to get people vaccinated. Her stories mainly deal with the smallpox vaccine and are quite interesting.

Another chapter connects SIDS deaths with the DPT vaccine and another connects tuberculosis with the TB vaccine. Oddly, she only briefly mentions pertussis vaccine and the large number of adverse reactions associated with it.

Because of the alarmist tone of this book, and the inaccurate and outdated information it contains, it is of limited value for use today. It is best read for the historical significance of past vaccine mishaps.

Available From:
PRISM (2). American Vegan Society (2).

Vaccinations Do Not Protect
Eleanor McBean, Ph.D., N.D. Austin, TX: The Health Library. 1980.
47 pp. (Republished in 1991 by Health Excellence Systems)

This is yet another book by Eleanor McBean. She wrote this book to briefly answer parents' questions while she was preparing her longer book, *Vaccination Condemned* (reviewed earlier in this Section). She has researched vaccination for 30 years.

She discusses the current vaccines as of 1980 and her strong opposition to them and to conventional medicine. She believes that vaccines cause disease instead of preventing it (e.g.; polio). She discards the germ theory.

Since she realizes that many of her readers oppose vaccination, she discusses legal exemptions in some detail. She includes an example of an exemption letter and sample state vaccination laws. She touches on international travel for the non-vaccinated.

Her language is very emotional. This book is not referenced.

Available From:
Out of print.

Section D

Current Research:
New Generation Vaccines

New vaccines currently under development use production techniques radically different from "conventional" vaccines. These new vaccines utilize the technologies of molecular biology, which includes genetic engineering. The first recombinant DNA vaccine to be used on a mass scale in the U.S. is the hepatitis B vaccine. Since we will be seeing more of these types of vaccines, and since most of the information available about them is highly technical, I'm including a lengthy introduction that contains short descriptions of the many different approaches to vaccine design now under investigation.

I collected the following descriptions from the books reviewed in this section. However, because I am trying to simplify highly technical material, which I admit, I at times had trouble understanding myself, I may not be completely accurate in my descriptions. I apologize for any errors, and should these be detected or pointed out to me, I will correct them in future editions.

New Methods of Vaccine Production Utilizing Molecular Biology

Recombinant DNA Procedures for Producing Vaccines

Antigens Harvested from Fermentation
In this approach, the gene in the disease organism responsible for producing the antigen is "cut out" and inserted into a foreign (host) organism (e.g., *E. coli*, yeasts, or animal cells). Once in this host cell

the gene "expresses" the antigen (i.e., the antigen multiples and grows) and then the antigen is "harvested" from the cell, purified, and made into a vaccine. The current hepatitis B vaccine is made this way using yeast cells.

Recombinant Live Vector Vaccines

These are vaccines which use a virus (e.g., *vaccinia*, polioviruses, adenoviruses, or herpes viruses), or a bacteria (e.g., *salmonella, BCG*) as a vector, which has the gene inserted which codes for the antigen from a disease organism. "Vector" means carrier. These viruses or bacteria "carry" the antigen gene into our cells when we are injected with the vaccine. If all goes as planned, the vector virus or bacteria "expresses" the gene in our body. This means that the gene does its work in producing the disease antigen in our body and our body then produces antibodies to the antigen. Since the only part of the disease organism actually used in the vaccine is the gene that codes for the antigen, it is hoped that adverse reactions will be greatly reduced. Vaccines under development using this approach include chicken pox, rabies, hepatitis A & B, Epstein-Barr, and HIV.

Naked DNA Vaccines, also called "DNA Vaccination"

Research on this type of vaccine is currently very popular. What this means is that the DNA coding of the disease antigens is used as a vaccine. Several ways of getting the DNA into the body are being experimented with. One is to place the DNA coding in a plasmid. A plasmid is a ring of DNA, usually of bacteria, that can replicate on their own. This would be inserted in the muscle. Another way under investigation is to coat gold beads with the DNA and shoot the beads under the skin. It is interesting to note that animal experiments have shown that while antibodies are created to these various DNA vaccines, researchers are still trying to understand how they actually function in the body.

Microencapsulated Vaccines

Antigens from the disease organism are placed in little capsules (called "copolymer microspheres") and administered orally. Early tests note higher antibody levels in mucosal surfaces, where our bodies first encounter disease organisms naturally, as compared to vaccines administered by shot. It is hoped to make these capsules time-release their contents so they provide their own booster doses. A new tetanus vaccine using this approach is in research.

Synthetic Polypeptide Vaccines, also called Peptide-based Vaccines

Peptides are amino acid chains. Amino acids are the building blocks of proteins. If a specific protein of the disease organism is determined to induce protective immunity in our bodies (meaning the protein is an antigen), then it may be possible to create by chemical synthesis, chains containing pure antigens. A vaccine for malaria using this approach is in clinical trials.

Anti-idiotypic Antibodies Vaccines

This approach is based on the "lock-and-key" theory of antibody function, which means that each antibody our body produces will fit into only one antigen in order to kill it; that is to say, we create disease specific antibodies. Antibodies are capable of stimulating the production of more antibodies. If a second antibody were somehow directed to attack the first antibody's mirror image, it would match the shape of the original antigen. These second antibodies or "surrogate antigens" are called anti-idiotypic antibodies. If these antibodies were used in vaccines, it is hoped that if the body were exposed to that disease organism the "surrogate antibodies" would bind to the organism and prevent infection.

The books reviewed below present the cutting edge of vaccine research. Unfortunately, they are highly technical, but I include one magazine article that is not so technical.

Modern Vaccinology
Edouard Kurstak, ed. NY: Plenum Medical Book Co. 1994. 397 pp.
ISBN 0-306-44820-3. Bibliography. Index.

This reference book is a collection of 18 chapters on current research and development of new vaccines written by doctors affiliated with various medical schools or vaccine manufacturers throughout the world. The editor, Edouard Kurstak, states in the introduction that what makes modern vaccinology different from past vaccinology is its use of new systems to deliver vaccines by using genetic engineering technology and recent progresses in molecular biology. New vaccines are being developed using the new genetic technology with an emphasis on the creation of more combined vaccines.

This book contains heavy technical jargon, some chapters more than others. One particularly interesting chapter describes the current combined vaccines DPT and MMR, their advantages and disadvantages, and also discusses the development of new generation, combined vaccines. Key factors that must be addressed in creating combined vaccines are: (1) biological compatibility of the antigens (i.e., making sure the immune responses do not interfere with each other); (2) pharmaceutical stability; (3) need and desirability; (4) technical feasibility; and (5) financial viability. Conventional combined vaccines have been of two types: inactivated (e.g., DPT) and live attenuated combined (e.g., MMR).

Difficulties with inactivated vaccines have been of two major types: (1) interference between the immune responses to the different antigens; and (2) physico-chemical incompatibilities between the components (e.g., preservatives, antigens, adjuvants, and excipients) making it difficult to have an effective, stable vaccine. The authors' state that the DPT vaccine has neither of these problems. Live attenuated combined vaccines have problems with the "take" of each of the components of the vaccine, for example, a person may produce a greater antibody response to one component antigen than to another. The authors feel this problem is best dealt with by limiting the upper limit of vaccines of this type combined together to four or five.

Development of new generation combined vaccines using the technology also being experimented with in developing monovalent", i.e., single-antigen, vaccines is examined. Major approaches to research described in this book are vector-combined vaccines, microencapsulated vaccines, naked DNA vaccines, synthetic polypeptide vaccines, and anti-idiotypic vaccines. These are described in the introduction to this Section. The last part of the book contains chapters detailing the progress in development of various new generation vaccines for specific diseases. These include an HIV vaccine, recombinant measles and recombinant pertussis vaccines.

I realize that few parents will read this book because of its technical difficulty. It is unfortunate that most material available on vaccine development is written solely for medical researchers. However, from this summary of the book it should be apparent that vaccine development has entered a whole new era, and we will be seeing new vaccines produced with these techniques in the coming years.

Available From:
Kluwer Academic Publishers (8).

The New Vaccines
Anna Aldovini and Richard A. Young. "Technology Review". January 1992. p. 25-31. Illus.

This magazine article explains in non-technical terms how the new vaccines are being developed using recombinant DNA technology. Anna Aldovini and Richard Young are doctors and researchers working on the development of an AIDS vaccine.

The authors describe how traditional vaccines are made and then compare this with how recombinant DNA vaccines are being made. Very simply explained, the gene, which contains instructions for producing an antigen, is isolated from a disease-causing virus. This gene is transplanted into a harmless virus or bacterium, which then reproduces the antigen. This harmless virus or bacterium is administered as a vaccine and the body is tricked into believing that the harmless virus or bacterium is the dangerous one and produces antibodies against the antigen. Genetically engineered vaccines are expected to produce fewer adverse reactions than traditional vaccines because the disease organism is not actually used in the vaccine. Other vaccines being researched for use with this technology are ones for Lyme disease, malaria, tetanus, measles, and AIDS.

Many detailed photographs and illustrations are sprinkled throughout. This easy-to-read article is highly recommended for those who want to understand the new vaccines.

Available From:
Check your local library for "Technology Review" magazine.

Strategies in Vaccine Design
Medical Intelligence Unit. Gordon L. Ada, ed. Georgetown, TX: R.G. Landes Co. 1994. 217 pp. ISBN 1-57059-094-X. Bibliography. Index.

This book, edited by Gordon L. Ada of the Australian National University Medical Research Department, examines the newest strategies in vaccine design, namely the use of molecular biology and genetic engineering to create more effective vaccines. It is written by immunologists for use by vaccinologists to explain the complex immune responses, which Dr. Ada believes many vaccinologists do not fully appreciate. Eleven papers are included written by various immunologists from around the world presenting their research on the immunology behind new generation vaccines.

In the preface, Dr. Ada explains the difference between the old ways of creating vaccines and the new ways. Basically, he says in the past research was done to balance the immunogenicity (i.e., the strength of the toxin, or antigen contained in the vaccine) against attenuation (attenuation lowers the ill effects of the disease organism so one doesn't catch it from the vaccine); thus, keeping the vaccine strong enough to create antibodies, but not too strong to make one sick. It was an imprecise operation and each batch of vaccine differed from each other (as all conventional vaccine batches still do). Now with advances in molecular biology, vaccine designers can create vaccines in which the antibody response can be precisely measured and a consistent response produced from vaccine batch to vaccine batch. Research in this area is growing by leaps and bounds and the papers contained in this volume present the latest information and opinions on new generation vaccines under development.

The papers are very technical; however, just an overview of the summaries reinforces the knowledge that current vaccine research is more focused on the details of cell-mediated immune response than could ever be done in the past.

A detailed picture is shown of how genetic engineering works, with at least one paper describing the genes of a virus and what functions they are known to perform and recommending "cut and paste" to create all sorts of combinations to use as vaccines. Each paper contains its own detailed bibliography of medical sources.

Available From:
Landes Bio Science (8).

Vaccine Research and Developments: Volume I
Wayne C. Koff and Howard R. Six, eds. NY: Marcel Dekker, Inc. 1992. 260 pp. ISBN 0-8247-8619-X. Index. Endnotes. Bibliography.

This is the first volume in a planned series on current vaccine research. From the list of contributors and the fact that one of the editors is from a pharmaceutical laboratory (Connaught) this appears to be a joint venture between private, government, and collegiate medical researchers. The papers contained here discuss the practical aspects of new vaccine development. Some of the papers are easier for the lay reader to understand than others, although you will be able to understand the introductions to each chapter.

Of particular interest is a section on clinical and legal aspects of vaccination. This section includes papers describing how vaccine clinical trials work and another on liability concerns for testing an AIDS vaccine. This paper includes background on vaccine liability and legal cases and information about the National Childhood Vaccine Injury Act of 1986. It is quite clear that vaccines can cause adverse effects; the problem, according to the author, is who is responsible and must pay damages.

Several of the papers are on research into the development of safer vaccines. Avenues being considered are: (1) testing different adjuvants to reduce adverse reactions (an adjuvant is a substance included in a vaccine to enhance the antibody response); (2) using "purer" antigens by "cutting" out the specific disease-causing antigen in a virus and discarding the rest of the virus (the "rest of the virus" is what usually causes the adverse reactions); and (3) production of acellular pertussis vaccine (which has now been approved by the FDA).

Another paper is on development of a contraceptive vaccine. One of the theories that the author describes is based on interrupting the hormonal balance so that the egg will reject any sperm that comes near it. However, one problem is how to make this effect temporary, so the woman will not be infertile for life. Another problem is how to make sure that the vaccine doesn't affect other organs in the body. Several different approaches are currently in research and clinical trials today. Messing around with basic human functions has important ethical and moral implications, something that the dry, technical language of this scientific paper completely ignores. (In other words, a contraceptive vaccine goes against Natural Law – God's Laws.)

This book is interesting reading. Everything is footnoted and each paper includes extensive bibliographies.

Available From:
Marcel Dekker, Inc. (8).

Section E

Books for Health Care Providers

The books reviewed in this Section are reference works written for pediatricians, family practitioners, nurses, and other health professionals who provide primary health care to children. You might be wondering why books written for health care providers are included in a guide directed mainly to parents. First of all, many health care providers use this book as a resource both for themselves and their patients. Secondly, it should interest parents to know what procedures are being recommended to health care providers by the CDC and other agencies regarding immunizations.

Epidemiology and Prevention of Vaccine-Preventable Diseases (The Pink Book)
William Atkinson, M.D., et. el., eds. Atlanta, GA: U.S. Dept. of Health and Human Services, CDC. Third edition. January 1996. 400 pp. No ISBN. Bibliography.

This manual, published by the CDC, presents a summary of government recommendations regarding childhood and adult vaccinations. This is the manual accompanying the telecourse of the same name. This course is presented periodically around the country. Although aimed at health care providers, the manual contains non-technical language making it easy reading for parents, as well. The authors give a much more thorough presentation of vaccination than any of the parent materials published by the CDC.

First, is an introductory chapter briefly explaining the principles of vaccination. This chapter is an excellent summary of the different classifications of vaccines dividing them by type (e.g., live, inactivated, conjugate, and recombinants) and briefly explaining how they differ. This is important information, as some authors critical of vaccinations tend to make these distinctions unclear.

There is a separate chapter on each of the following vaccines: diphtheria, tetanus, pertussis, polio, measles, mumps, rubella, varicella (chickenpox), hepatitis B, Hib, influenza, and pneumonia. Each chapter covers the following points: (1) a description of the disease including clinical features, complications, and how to make a correct diagnosis; (2) a recent history of the disease occurrence in the U.S. with graphs from both before and after vaccinations started; (3) a short history of the development of each vaccine and how it is manufactured; (4) adverse reactions and contraindications; and (5) vaccine storage and handling. An important feature of each section are vaccine timetables that provide information on the standard immunization schedule, but also timetables for those whose immunizations are delayed past the usual ages. This is important for parents to know who delay immunizations for whatever reason. Information is also provided that explains which shots can and can not be given together and the minimum spacing required between different shots of the same vaccine or between different vaccines.

Half of the book consists of a variety of appendices. These include: (1) a copy of the ACIP general recommendations on immunizations; (2) the *Standards for Pediatric Immunization Practices* (reviewed in Section A.2); (3) documents on adult immunization; (4) a listing of state immunization offices; (5) samples of the CDC Vaccine Information Statements (VIS's, reviewed in Section A.2); and (6) information on the National Vaccine Injury Compensation Program.

For doctors, this is a good basic reference manual on vaccines and their correct administration. For parents, this book provides detailed, clearly presented information in easy to understand terms, and is especially helpful in explaining the different types of vaccines and timetables for vaccine administration. The fifth edition is now available and covers more vaccines. The manual is no longer free, but you can download a free copy (it's big) from the CDC website. It is not footnoted, although a bibliography is provided.

Available From:
CDC (1).

Immunization Delivery: A Complete Guide
John D. Grabenstein, MS Pharm. Ed.M, FASHP, FRSH. St. Louis, MO:
Facts and Comparisons. 1997. 183 pp. ISBN 1-57439-020-1. Index.
References.

This book is a guide for pharmacists, nurses, and doctors who want
to help boost immunization rates, especially among adults. Dr.
Grabenstein is a clinical pharmacist with the U.S. Army Medical
Dept. He wrote this book in his capacity as a private citizen. Dr.
Grabenstein is very concerned about promoting the use of vaccines.
He encourages all medical personnel to use every opportunity to
locate and encourage people to be vaccinated. This book covers
childhood vaccines, but Dr. Grabenstein emphasizes adult vaccines.
Since adults are not required by law to receive vaccines, they are
less likely to ask or seek them. Dr. Grabenstein believes that all
medical personnel should be aggressive in asking and encouraging
high-risk adult groups to be vaccinated, especially with influenza
and pneumococcal vaccines.

Dr. Grabenstein includes a detailed chapter on immunization
documentation. He states that for adults especially, their medical
records may be scattered among many health providers and it may
be quite difficult to determine what vaccines they have already
received and which to recommend. He advocates for centralized
immunization documentation, in other words, a computerized
immunization registry. A whole chapter is devoted to legal issues
and liability. He states that most states have laws protecting providers against malpractice suits involving vaccine delivery, especially
for required vaccines. Only negligence or wrongful acts are sometimes not covered under these protections.

Separate chapters directed to pharmacists, nurses, and doctors
explain ways each can become more effective vaccine advocates
and increase immunization rates in their communities. Another
chapter covers ways health providers can get reimbursed for offering free vaccines through the Vaccines for Children Program (VCP).

This book is footnoted with material from medical journals and
government reports. He includes a list of organizations that may
offer assistance in promoting vaccines. Overall, this is a succinct
and useful book for those who wish to promote the use of vaccines,
especially for adults.

Available From:
Out of print.

Immunization: Precautions and Contraindications

George C. Kassianos, M.D. London: Blackwell Scientific Publications.
1994. 222 pp. ISBN 0-86542-887-5. Index.

George Kassianos is a Family Practitioner in Great Britain. This
book is written for British pediatricians and other health care workers as a reference guide for childhood vaccines, adult vaccines, and
vaccines for those traveling abroad.

Although the subtitle is "Precautions and Contraindications"
and Dr. Kassianos does list these for each vaccine, he is very
conservative in what he allows as contraindications and stresses the
need for doctors to dispel the "myth" of certain medical conditions
as valid contraindications. This is similar to the current push by the
CDC to eliminate "false" contraindications. For example, Dr.
Kassianos states that a child with a stable neurological condition
should be immunized with pertussis. However, the CDC recommends in its *Guide to Contraindications to Childhood Vaccinations*
(reviewed in Section B.1) that the child "may be vaccinated" and
this should be discussed and evaluated on an individual basis with
the doctor. Dr. Kassianos also downplays adverse reactions associated with vaccines, especially pertussis.

You might wonder why I am including a review of a book written for a British audience. Well, I find it interesting to make a
comparison between their childhood vaccine schedule and ours. The
British adopted an accelerated immunization schedule for infants in
1990. The doses of vaccine which are administered in the U.S. at
two, four, and six months of age were changed in Britain to two,
three, and four months of age. These include DTP, Hib, and polio.
MMR is given at the same time as here (12 to 15 months). In Britain
only three doses of DTP are given. There are no fourth and fifth
doses as in the U.S. (at 12 to 18 months and 4 to 6 years of age),
instead a DT shot is given at 4 to 5 years of age in Britain. A fourth
dose of polio vaccine is also given at 4 to 5 years of age, the same as
here.

This vaccine schedule change was part of a large nation-wide program to increase immunization rates in Britain, which has been quite successful due to monetary incentives given to health care providers if they achieve certain minimum immunization rates (70%) and additional payments if they achieve 90% or higher immunization rates within their practices. Dr. Kassianos does not mention this aspect of Britain's immunization program in his book, but you can find a summary of it in the IOM report, *Overcoming Barriers to Immunization* (reviewed in Section G.2).

Dr. Kassianos describes each of the childhood and adult vaccines, noting contraindications, adverse reactions, a description of the disease and of the vaccine, and to whom and when the vaccine should be administered. He also describes vaccines for those traveling abroad (e.g., yellow fever, typhoid, cholera, malaria, and others).

This is a basic reference book reflecting the medical community's views on vaccination in Britain.

Available From:
Out of print.

Pocket Guide to Vaccination and Prophylaxis
Hal B. Jenson, M.D. Philadelphia, PA: W. B. Saunders Co. 1999. 313 pp. ISBN 0-7216-7993-5. Index. Bibliography.

As the title suggests, this is a succinct guide for health professionals on vaccination and prophylaxis. It is written by Hal Jenson, Chief of the Division of Pediatric Infectious Diseases at the University of Texas Health Science Center. Dr. Jenson combines together the recommendation and guidelines produced by the Advisory Committee on Immunization Practices of the CDC (ACIP), the American Academy of Pediatrics (AAP), the American College of Physicians (ACP), the American Academy of Family Physicians (AAFP), the American College of Obstetricians and Gynecologists (ACOG), the American Medical Association (AMA), and the Infectious Diseases Society of America (IDSA). Where their recommendations differ, he notes so in the text and in the many tables contained in the book. This helps the clinician, who may be swamped with reports from these many organizations, to keep all the information straight. Dr. Jenson uses tables whenever possible to present material in an easily accessible fashion.

The book is divided into two main sections. The first section deals with vaccination. Dr. Jenson covers all vaccines available in the U.S., including vaccines recommended for children, adults, health care workers, and people who are immuno-compromised. He describes each vaccine and when and to whom it should be administered. He also lists contraindications and noncontraindications. He explains which adverse events following vaccination require mandatory reporting, and which others are voluntary. He includes the most recent National Vaccine Injury Compensation Program (NVICP) Vaccine Injury Table for use in filing for compensation from the government for vaccine injuries. Included are detailed explanations of the type of injuries that are and are not covered under the NVICP. There is a table that nicely summarizes the findings of the two IOM reports, *Adverse Effects of Pertussis and Rubella Vaccines* and *Adverse Events Associated with Childhood Vaccines: Evidence Bearing on Causality* (both reviewed in Section B), on adverse events associated with vaccines. Vaccines and prophylaxis for the international traveler are explained in detail. Also included are tips and suggestions for avoiding disease.

The second half of the book covers prophylaxis. Prophylaxis is a health measure designed to preserve health and prevent the spread of infectious disease. Covered here are guidelines for handling possible exposure to rabies, tetanus, pertussis, hepatitis B, and other diseases. Also covered is perinatal prophylaxis such as Group B streptococcal infection, which can possibly be transmitted to an infant at birth. Prophylaxis for dental procedures, other surgeries, and HIV are explained as well.

Dr. Jenson includes a bibliography containing all the reports that he draws his summaries from. He also lists vaccination resources including books (textbooks directed to medical professionals), websites, VAERS, vaccine manufacturers, immune globulin manufacturers, and travel information hotlines. Overall, this is a very handy guide combining a large volume of material into an easy to use format. Dr. Jenson notes that since information and recommendations are always changing, you can access updates on the

University of Texas Health Science Center's website: www.vaccine. uthsca.edu. This makes the book an even more valuable resource.

Available From:
Elsevier Health Science (8).

Report of the Committee on Infectious Diseases (The Red Book)
Committee on Infectious Diseases Staff, American Academy of Pediatrics. Elk Grove Village, IL: American Academy of Pediatrics. 1994. 23rd Edition. 687 pp. ISBN 0-910761-48-5.

Every three years the Committee on Infectious Diseases of the American Academy of Pediatrics (AAP) publishes its report on the current status of infectious diseases. The report is referred to as the "Red Book". Its intended audience is pediatricians.

Included in this report are the committee's recommendations concerning childhood vaccines. Childhood diseases are described with special emphasis on diagnosis and explanation of the course of the disease. Ways of prevention are listed and this includes immunizations. Adverse reactions and contraindications are also addressed.

Not much is allowed in the way of contraindications. For example, they state that it is not considered a contraindication for receiving pertussis vaccine if the child has a family history of seizures (the CDC agrees with this). If the child has a personal history of seizures, it is considered a reason for delaying only; the child's status should be reevaluated at each subsequent visit and if no further seizures are expected then the DPT shot can be given. Their view is that as few children as possible should be denied the benefits of vaccines. Of course, as the authors point out, children do not usually develop a history of seizures until after they have already received their first DPT shot, as it is unusual for a two month old baby to have a prior history of convulsions. They further state that since most convulsions that occur after a vaccine are associated with a fever, they are only "febrile convulsions", and therefore not serious and not to be concerned about. A resulting seizure disorder is not considered a reaction from a vaccine, but a pre-existing, undetected neurological condition that was "brought out" by the vaccine.

The position of the AAP is to vaccinate everyone because they strongly believe that the benefits far outweigh the risks. This book is not footnoted. The 25th edition will be available in May 2000.

Available From:
American Academy of Pediatrics (2).

Standards for Pediatric Immunization Practices
National Vaccine Advisory Committee. Atlanta, GA: Centers for Disease Control and Prevention. Adopted 1992. 31 pp.

This booklet briefly outlines 18 standards for pediatric immunization practices recommended by the National Vaccine Advisory Committee (NVAC). These standards have been approved by the U. S. Public Health Service and endorsed by the American Academy of Pediatrics (AAP), the Advisory Committee on Immunization Practices (ACIP), and the American Nurses Association (ANA), among others. This booklet is addressed to health care professionals, but parents will find it interesting, as well.

These standards were issued to help realize the year 2000 objective of 90% immunization of all two-year-olds. Some readers may recall hearing news reports in 1993 that the vaccination rate of children under two years of age was 50% - 60% (different news reports gave different percentages). Because of mandatory vaccination for school age children and many preschool programs, percentage rates for these older children are 90% to 100%.

The 18 standards stress the need to take advantage of every opportunity to vaccinate (e.g., coordinate with other appointments, or inquire about vaccination status of children when parents visit the doctor), and destroy the barriers to vaccination (e.g., extend clinic hours, allow walk-ins, offer free vaccines, allow trained non-medical personnel to vaccinate, or reduce the physical exam time). It lists what the ACIP and AAP agree are true contraindications and precautions for each vaccine. It also lists "not true" contraindications, because of concerns that doctors are accepting these as true contraindications and missing an opportunity to vaccinate.

Included in the 18 standards are references to the National Vaccine Injury Compensation Program and the importance of following this law. This includes providing patients with information about risks and benefits, completely recording the vaccine data in patients' files, and reporting adverse reactions to health authorities.

Whether you support vaccination or are critical of vaccinations these standards should concern you. Why? Because the obligations created by the National Vaccine Injury Compensation Program may come in conflict with the desire to hurriedly immunize as many children as possible by the year 2000. How can true contraindications be accurately assessed if shots are administered in assembly-line fashion, with a minimal physical exam by non-medical personnel?

Available From:
National Immunization Program (1). Free.

Use and Standardization of Combined Vaccines
Developments in Biological Standardization Series, Vol. 65
International Association of Biological Standardization, ed. Basel, Switzerland: S. Karger. 1986. 284 pp. ISBN 3-8055-4461-8. Index. Bibliography.

This book contains the proceedings of a symposium organized by the International Association of Biological Standardization (IABS) held in Amsterdam in December 1985. Seven sessions were held each on different combined vaccines.

These papers focus on clinical applications of vaccines, their efficacy ("efficacy" means how well they work) and safety, and how to boost immunization rates using combined vaccines and simultaneously administered vaccines (e.g., DPT, OPV, and MMR all at one visit). Researchers from Europe and the U.S. presented papers explaining the vaccination situation in their countries. The main problem is determining the best age to vaccinate versus increased/decreased efficacy rates, as well as how different vaccines simultaneously administered effect efficacy.

I include summaries of two papers that should be of interest to parents. One paper from Switzerland evaluated the trials of a new MMR vaccine that may prove to cause fewer allergic reactions than the one in current use. The current MMR vaccine is cultured in chicken embryos and anyone with a severe allergy to eggs is cautioned about receiving it. The new vaccine being tested is produced in human diploid cells and therefore, contains no chicken protein or antibiotics, which may cause allergic reactions. (The question to ask, however, is what is the source for the human diploid cells? Other vaccines, which I have researched, which use human diploid cell lines have obtained them from aborted fetuses.)

Another paper, this one from doctors in Philadelphia, presents the results of clinical trials on vaccine efficacy following different combinations of simultaneously administered vaccines (e.g., MMR, OPV, and DTP given together). Although participant numbers were quite small (only in the hundreds); no difference in rate of adverse effects or vaccine efficacy was noted when all these vaccines were given at the same time, instead of at time intervals.

The overall conclusion of the symposium was that combined vaccines reduce the number of doctor visits needed to complete the recommended vaccinations, thus resulting in higher vaccination levels without an increase in adverse reactions or lowering of vaccine efficacy.

Available From:
Out of print.

Vaccines
Stanley A. Plotkin, M.D. and Edward A. Mortimer, M.D., eds. Philadelphia, PA: W. B. Saunders Co. 1994. Second edition. 996 pp. ISBN 0-7216-6584-5. Index. Endnotes. Bibliography.

This is a detailed reference manual to help doctors and all interested people better understand vaccines and their historical context. Most of the 56 contributors to the second edition are professors at various medical schools.

Individual chapters are devoted to each of the childhood vaccines in current use. New vaccines in development are also included (e.g., AIDS, and hepatitis A), as well as vaccines for tropical diseases, such as yellow fever and cholera. It is not overly technical, though a basic understanding of immunology terms would be helpful.

The chapters for each vaccine are patterned the same. First, the historical background of the disease is presented and a clinical description is given. Next, is a detailed description of the virus or bacterium and how it was found and isolated. A correct diagnosis of the disease is explained. The epidemiology (where and how it occurs throughout the world) is discussed and its relevance as a public health problem. Passive immunization and description of the available forms and how they work is explained. Active immunization, which includes a history of the particular vaccine strains and their development, and specific dosage information and route of administration (orally, subcutaneously, or intramuscularly) are detailed. The actual production of the vaccine and its degree of stability is described. Immune responses, the possibility of catching the disease after vaccination and protective effects of the vaccine are analyzed, as well as how long immunity lasts. Many of the studies they include give conflicting information on how long immunity is conferred. Contraindications are listed. These are conservative. Side effects and complications are discussed, though severe complications are considered rare.

Epidemiological results of vaccination are discussed at the end of each chapter. They all show that vaccines have contributed to a large decrease in incidences of that particular disease. (Statistics are mostly from this century, or since WWII.) New to the second edition are chapters on the regulation and testing of vaccines, new vaccine technologies, and vaccination laws and liability.

Many graphs and tables are strewn throughout. Many studies are presented. The lack of studies on long-term effects is quite evident and noted matter-of-factly throughout. Every chapter is liberally footnoted and all chapters include extensive journal article endnotes. The book is well organized making it easy to look up facts; for example, finding the date that measles vaccine was first approved for use is easy to locate.

If I could have only one authoritative reference book on vaccines, this would be it. I have used it repeatedly in checking the accuracy of other authors' research. For parents it provides historically accurate information about the development of each vaccine strain, which is sometimes presented in a confused manner or inaccurately in other non-technical vaccination books. Due to the high price (around $200), few parents, if any, will be able to afford to purchase this text; however, they should be able to find a copy at a medical library or request it through interlibrary loan at their local library. The third edition was published in 1999 and covers the newest vaccines.

Available From:
Elsevier Health Science (8). The third edition has 1230 pp. ISBN 0-7216-7443-7. The 4th edition is due out in Oct. 2003.

Section F

Legal Exemptions

If after making your informed decision about vaccinations for your child, you decide to give your child the vaccines either following CDC or AAP recommendations, you do not have to be concerned about your child being accepted into school. However, if your decision is not to vaccinate your child with any or all vaccines, then unfortunately, because of compulsory immunization laws, you must obtain a legal exemption to enroll your child in public school (and most private schools, too).

The books reviewed in this section give parents advice to help them better understand how to obtain a legal exemption and reduce the fear or intimidation they may feel. Most of the books reviewed in Sections A and B also contain chapters on obtaining exemptions that are very helpful. See Resources (3) for the names of organizations, individuals, and lawyers who may be able to help.

It should be noted that because of the political climate of the 1990's, legal exemptions were challenged in many states by health officials, schools and in state legislatures. Several states have had "battles" in recent years over abolishing or adding philosophical exemption clauses. It is imperative if you want to obtain an exemption, or currently have one, to keep a close watch on the legislative situation in your state. In March 2000, Iowans almost lost its religious exemption, but concerned citizens who supported religious freedoms flooded the Iowa legislature with phone calls and email and the religious exemption was restored. Several state and national vaccine organizations provide up-to-date information on legal exemptions and actively lobby government officials about exemptions. You may want to consider joining one or more of these groups (see under Legal Exemptions in Resources).

Attorney James Filenbaum has written an article on obtaining legal exemptions for the Spring 2000 issue of "Innovations" magazine. He has given me permission to include an excerpted version of that article here, which should prove informative for those seeking a religious exemption.

YOUR RIGHTS TO AVOID IMMUNIZATIONS
By: James R. Filenbaum, Esq.
Excerpted from *Innovation,* Spring 2000 issue

A great deal of concern regarding immunizations has recently been given considerable media attention. While many people are now looking at alternative information sources as to the choice of whether to have their children immunized, their rights are often not clearly explained. As an attorney who has represented many people who have secured exemptions from immunizations, and has won the leading Federal Court cases which have expanded peoples' rights to claim exemptions from immunizations, I have become particularly familiar with this area of the law.

Most States only allow an exemption from immunizations for children attending school based upon religious beliefs or by a licensed physician signing a certificate indicating that the immunizations are contraindicated. Some States have taken a more liberal approach in the enactment of statutes that allow for children to be admitted into school attendance based upon the parents' request for an exemption.

Securing the medical exemption is extremely difficult since only those criteria approved by the American Medical Association and American Academy of Pediatrics as contraindication for each immunization are considered valid by school districts or Health Departments. Therefore, requests for exemptions for medical reasons are extremely limited.

Valid claims for exemption from immunizations based upon religious beliefs now encompass PERSONAL religious beliefs. This is a much broader base than was possible before we won several landmark cases. A great number of people fail to utilize this right to a religious exemption because they view religion in traditional terms and do not feel the exemption can apply to them because they are not members of a specific church, such as the Christian Scientists.

Religion goes far beyond simple membership in a church, attendance of services, adherence to prescribed dogma, or participation in various rituals. While an exact definition of what would constitute a "religious belief" varies depending upon what purpose is being applied to the use of the word "religion in", pursuing a claim for a religious exemption from immunizations the standard which must be considered is that which is established by the United States Supreme Court. Therefore, in adherence to the First Amendment of the United States Constitution guarantee of freedom of religion, the test in determining whether a belief constitutes a "religious belief" sufficient to qualify for the religious exemption from immunizations, is whether the adherents' beliefs and faiths occupy a place in their lives parallel to that filled by the orthodox belief in God held by others; or any other "sincere religious beliefs which are based upon a power or being, or upon a faith to which all else is subordinate or upon which all else is ultimately dependent." *U.S. Vs. Seeger, 380 U.S. 163 (1965), Sherr and Levy vs. Northport East-Northport Union Free School district, 672 F.Supp. 81, (E.D.N.Y. 1987).*

The right to claim exemption from immunization based on religious beliefs is available to all persons who hold religious beliefs against immunization regardless of what any state statute may say regarding the necessity for membership in any particular religious group or church.

The first amendment to the U.S. Constitution prohibits states from discriminating between people based on their religious beliefs. If there is any state law that allows for exemption based on religious beliefs, it is available to all those people who hold religious beliefs against immunization even if their beliefs are personal and unique to them alone.

Dangers of Compulsory Immunizations: How to Avoid Them Legally
Tom Finn, Esq. Port Richey, FL: Family Fitness Press. 1983. 53 pp.
No ISBN. Footnotes. Resources.

Tom Finn is a trial lawyer specializing in health freedom issues, including combating compulsory immunization laws. In this book, Mr. Finn briefly covers the history of the polio vaccine, compulsory vaccination laws, and the current medical controversy.

He describes the three ways to claim an exemption from vaccinations: religious, medical, and personal beliefs. The only one that he discusses in depth is religious exemption. In this area, he concludes that the legal battle rests on the state's interests to protect all citizens against communicable diseases, versus the individual's

religious freedom. In most past cases the state has won, but Mr.
Finn believes that this will change, as risks of epidemics wane and
state's interests arguments diminish in strength.

Mr. Finn, however, does say that a person may try to challenge
the vaccination laws on the right to privacy law. This includes the
right to control one's own body and make fundamental decisions
about one's own life. According to Mr. Finn, as of 1983, this has not
been successfully used to combat compulsory vaccination laws.

This book is footnoted and documented mostly with court cases.

Available From:
Out of print.

Vaccination: A Guide to Informed Choice
Section I: Facts. Section II: Rights.
Sharon Kimmelman, ed. NY: Vaccination Alternatives. Nov. 1997.
8 ½" x 11" stapled pages in two separate sections. Section I: 32 pp.
Section II: 62 pp. No ISBN. Note: Updated as needed.

Sharon Kimmelman wants parents to realize that they do have a
choice and should inform themselves about vaccination. She makes
it clear in the brief introduction to Section I that she is completely
opposed to mandatory vaccination. Sharon Kimmelman is director
of "Vaccination Alternatives", a New York City based vaccination
organization, whose main purpose is to provide information to
parents so they can make an informed choice. While she treats
vaccination and health in general in Section I, Section II is devoted
to obtaining legal exemptions and comprises the bulk of this guide.

Most of Section I contains excerpts from newspaper articles and
reports from alternative health newsletters. Several articles attempt
to connect AIDS with vaccination. She supports the view that
toxemia (buildup of toxic wastes in the body) is the basic cause of
disease.

Section II is for those who have decided not to vaccinate and
want to know their legal rights. It is divided into five parts.

Part one is on the new baby. Ms. Kimmelman relays the questions and concerns that new parents experience when deciding
whether or not to vaccinate their infant. Her intent is to get parents

to think differently about health and disease by questioning our drug-enamored, germ hunting medical system in favor of a health-promoting, immune-enhancing approach.

Part two is about children entering school. It explains legal exemptions. She answers common questions parents have who are worried about confronting school officials. She alleges that school officials are bullied by the Department of Health into denying exemptions for students. Several newspaper stories are clipped of parents winning court cases in New York that allowed them a religious exemption for their children.

Part three concerns students entering college. Ms. Kimmelman's strong bias against the medical establishment shows here. She believes that college students are frightened into getting vaccinated without being informed about the availability of exemptions. Her book is one of the few books I have read that covers college-age vaccinations.

Part four is on travel abroad. She reprints an informative article from the National Health Federation's "Immunization Kit". This article is on quarantine procedures for an individual who has returned to the U.S. from an infected country.

Part five is an important section. Ms. Kimmelman, using New York vaccination laws as an example, gives specific guidelines for applying for a medical, religious, or personal exemption. She includes sample exemption letters for claiming a religious exemption.

This guide provides valuable information to parents. It is especially applicable to New York State residents. She also has sample exemption letters based on New Jersey and Connecticut state laws, just request them when ordering.

Neither Section is footnoted or documented.

Available From:
Sharon Kimmelman is no longer active as of Dec. 2001 and her guide is no longer available. The Coalition for Informed Choice (1) issues a similar guide for NYS residents only.

**Vaccine Exemptions: A State-by-State Summary of Legal
Exemptions to "Mandatory" Vaccine Laws**
Santa Fe, NM: New Atlantean Press. 1995. 16 pp. ISBN 1-881217-07-8.

This little pamphlet contains what the subtitle says, a state-by-state
summary of legal exemptions to mandatory vaccine laws. Mr. Neil
Miller, who has written three other books on vaccinations (see
reviews in Sections A.1, B.1 and C), has compiled this summary to
aid parents who may be moving to a new state and are interested in
knowing the legal exemptions there. I found it useful just comparing
the wide variety of wording used in each state's laws, especially
regarding religious exemptions and philosophical exemptions.

Mr. Miller states that this book contains summaries of each
state's immunization laws. What he means, is he includes the actual
wording for the legal exemptions that each state allows and the part
of the law explaining which vaccinations are required for school
admittance. Consult a copy of your state code at the public library.

At the end of the book is a chart summarizing the types of
exemptions allowed in each state. Mr. Miller notes whether a certain
state requires adherence or membership in a recognized church
opposed to vaccinations to qualify for a religious exemption, or if it
allows personal religious beliefs to qualify. He includes a sample
affidavit to use for a religious or philosophical exemption if your
state does not have a standard form or certificate.

Overall, a useful and informative guide.

Available From:
New Atlantean Press (8).

Your Personal Guide to Immunization Exemptions
Grace Girdwain. Pittsburgh, PA: Dorrance Publishing Co., Inc. 2000.
34 pp. ISBN 0-8059-3319-0. Resources.

The purpose of this book is to show parents how to obtain legal
exemptions to vaccinations. Ms. Girdwain is director of Special
Human Rights Services and has advised parents for over 25 years on
their legal right to obtain vaccination exemptions. She previously

wrote a small booklet on obtaining legal exemptions which is now part of the book *The Immune Trio*, reviewed in Section B.3.

Ms. Girdwain gives advice on filling out exemption forms and dealing with school and health officials. She briefly discusses medical and religious exemptions and even provides samples of exemption letters. She does not discuss philosophical exemptions, although she does provide a sample exemption letter. She updated the book in 1999 and added a chapter on divorce and child custody issues pertaining to exemptions.

A great resource for those who are not vaccinating.

Available From:
Dorrance Publishing Co. (3). Global Vaccine Awareness League (1). Koren Publications (8). Special Human Rights Services (3).

Section G

Federal Vaccination Programs

Section G.1: The National Childhood Vaccine Injury Act of 1986

When the National Childhood Vaccine Injury Act of 1986 (NCVIA) was enacted it established the National Vaccine Injury Compensation Program (NVICP). This program provides for a no-fault system to compensate people who have died or suffered permanent disabilities resulting from vaccines. The NVICP went into effect on October 1, 1988. Vaccine manufacturers welcomed the relief from lawsuits. Parents were glad that the government was willing to take financial responsibility for children whose lives were damaged by mandatory vaccinations.

Unfortunately, in the decade since this program went into effect, what was supposed to be a quick and "painless" way to receive financial compensation, has turned into years of court proceedings and grief for many parents who have tried to use this program. The Vaccine Injury Table, which contains the type of injuries allowed, has been modified and tightened over the years making it harder to obtain compensation. To qualify for compensation, one must show that a "table injury" occurred within the specified time period, prove the vaccine caused the injury, or prove the vaccine aggravated a pre-existing condition. Since it is easier to show a table injury, this is the choice usually selected. However, if the court can show that the injury was not related to the vaccine, the claim will be denied, even if it is a table injury. Because of this, the "no fault" process has instead become a highly adversarial one. The National Vaccine Information Center (NVIC) has followed the NVICP closely and can offer parents advice. The Advisory Commission on Childhood Vaccines meets quarterly to advise the Secretary of Health and Human services on the NVICP and recommend changes to the

Vaccine Injury Table. The commission is composed of three health care professionals, three members of the public, and three attorneys.

If you choose to seek damages through this program, you must first waive your right to sue the vaccine manufacturer or vaccine provider. You can request claim forms, the current Vaccine Injury Table, or copies of the legislation from the Division of Vaccine Injury Compensation listed in Resources (6). One of the publications reviewed below discusses the NCVIA.

The NCVIA also established the National Vaccine Program Office (NVPO). The NVPO coordinates and provides direction for vaccine development, testing, licensing, production, procurement, distribution, delivery, and continued evaluation of vaccines already in use in the U.S. It operates within the Office of the Assistant Secretary for Health, part of the U.S. Dept. of Health and Human Services. In order to do these activities the NVPO was to issue an annual National Vaccine Plan (NVP) to be approved by Congress. The Reagan Administration did not support the NVPO and therefore did not fund it, so no annual NVPs were written during the Reagan and Bush years. The first, and so far only, NVP was written in 1994. A summary of it is included here.

Disease Prevention through Vaccine Development and Immunization: The U.S. National Vaccine Plan - 1994
The National Vaccine Program Office. March 1994. 127 pp.

This plan presents the four goals of the National Vaccine Program Office (NVPO) for increasing the vaccination rate among all age groups. These goals were developed by the National Vaccine Advisory Committee (NVAC) whose duty it is to advise the NVPO. The NVPO was created in 1986 as part of the NCVIA. The NVPO was supposed to develop a National Vaccine Plan (NVP) on an annual basis; however, this is the first and only plan to date.

The goals of the NVPO are: (1) development of new and im-proved vaccines; (2) optimizing safety and effectiveness of vaccines; (3) better educating of the public and health professionals about the benefits of vaccinations; and (4) better use of existing vaccines. To attain these goals numerous strategies and actions are rec-ommended. Most of the strategies reflect what is contained in the

CDC's *Standards of Pediatric Immunization Practices* (reviewed in Section E) and in the report *Overcoming Barriers to Immunization* (reviewed in Section G.2), that is, take advantage of every opportunity to vaccinate. The goals of the Childhood Immunization Initiative (CII) are included in the NVP. (The CII is explained in the introduction to Section G.2.) Other strategies include federally subsidizing the cost of vaccines, enforcing vaccination laws, streamlining the FDA licensing process for new vaccines, and stockpiling vaccines for emergency use.

Available From:
NVPO (1).

Immunization Dice: A 20th Century Fund Paper
Michael Brody. NY: Priority Press Publications. 1987. 80p.
ISBN 0-87078-211-8. Footnotes.

The Twentieth Century Fund is a non-profit research foundation founded in 1919 which presents analyses of economic, political, and social issues. This report by journalist Michael Brody, who has experience covering product liability issues, explains what the Fund believes is a "vaccine crisis". This crisis is the result of large payments in lawsuit settlements in the late 1970's and early 1980's against vaccine manufacturers that led several vaccine manufacturers to stop making vaccines altogether, resulting in a shortage of available vaccines. The 1986 National Childhood Vaccine Injury Act (NCVIA) had just been passed prior to the writing of this report, and Mr. Brody discusses the impact that this no-fault government insurance system may have on the "vaccine crisis".

Mr. Brody begins by stating that prior to the passage of the 1986 Act, vaccine manufacturers made little profit on the sales of their vaccines while worrying about potential large sum lawsuits brought against them for vaccine damages. He continues by stating that "more than 100 children die or suffer brain damage or paralysis each year" as a result of vaccine reactions from all childhood vaccines, but that this is "accepted as the tragic but unavoidable price of saving others". He believes that most, if not all, of the vaccine damage lawsuits do not reflect any wrongful manufacturing by the vaccine maker, but instead is just the price a few individuals must pay to save the lives of millions of others. Therefore, vaccine damage will continue to occur, and unless the current practice of hugh million dollar lawsuits isn't changed soon, Mr. Brody contends, no manufacturer will be left to make vaccines. This is the "vaccine crisis".

Mr. Brody includes a chapter on the recent history of tort laws, that is, laws dealing with injuries from products, and how changes in these laws since the 1960's have resulted in the current rash of large monetary settlement cases in all areas of product manufacturing. He explains how federal and state governments have acted to pass or attempted to pass legislation to control the misuse of these laws. He then focuses specifically on the development of the 1986 NCVIA. Mr. Brody's main concern is that if the NCVIA, which at the time it was passed only covered damages due from the then eight childhood vaccines, did not allow for the inclusion of any newly developed vaccines, this omission would prevent vaccine manufacturers from developing new vaccines, since they could not be assured that liability would be covered by the government and not rest on their shoulders. (The law has since been changed so that Hib, hepatitis B, and chickenpox have been added to the program and any new vaccine recommended by the CDC for universal administration to children will be added.) Mr. Brody states that vaccine companies make very little profit from vaccines because of the high cost of liability insurance and lawsuits. Since they provide a "life or death" product of which 50% is sold to government health care providers and mandated by state laws, Mr. Brody believes that the federal government should shoulder the burden of liability. Mr. Brody is especially concerned that the development of an AIDS vaccine could be delayed or stopped altogether because manufacturers may be faced with lawsuits that they could not pay.

Mr. Brody is excited about the production of genetically engineered vaccines, which he believes will produce far fewer adverse reactions than the conventional vaccines, thus reducing the number of lawsuits and liability worries of the manufacturers. But he does note that no vaccine is 100% safe and even these new genetically engineered ones may create some adverse reactions.

Mr. Brody wrote this report in 1987 before he could see the effect of the 1986 Act. Therefore, he includes little critique of the

NCVIA, but hopes that it will solve the "vaccine crisis". (It would be interesting to know what he thinks of the NCVIA today). This book is of most interest for the light it sheds on the history of tort laws and specifically on the development of the NCVIA.

Available From:
The Brookings Institution (8).

Section G.2

The Childhood Immunization Initiative of 1993

On August 10, 1993, Congress passed the Comprehensive Child Immunization Act of 1993 also called the Childhood Immunization Initiative (CII) as part of the Omnibus Budget Reconciliation Act. It went into effect on October 1, 1994. The aim of the CII was to eliminate childhood cases of six vaccine-preventable diseases: diphtheria, Hib, measles, polio, rubella, and tetanus, and to significantly reduce cases of pertussis, hepatitis B, and mumps by 1996. To accomplish this aim the CII has worked to increase vaccination rates for two-year-old children to 90% by 1996. Specific activities included increased funding for Immunization Action Plans (IAPS). IAPs are plans developed by states and major urban areas to increase the immunization rate of two-year-olds. Funds were made available through the CDC beginning in 1992 to increase these programs. Other activities of the CII include: (1) improving disease surveillance; (2) providing accurate measurement of immunization coverage; (3) coordinating immunization activities among federal departments, agencies, and private organizations; and (4) encouraging the development of safer and more effective vaccines with an emphasis on developing more combination vaccines. The National Vaccine Program Office (NVPO), established in 1986, is responsible for overseeing all aspects of the CII. The CDC has been placed in charge of the operational aspects. This includes the administering of major grant programs (e.g., for states to implement computerized tracking systems of immunization status, see Section G.3 for more details), providing technical assistance to public health departments, and conducting disease surveillance.

Media attention has been focused primarily on the portion of the CII called the Vaccines for Children Program (VCP), which provides free vaccines to eligible children. Under this program, the federal government purchases vaccines in bulk from vaccine manufacturers and distributes them to states free of charge. Each state is in charge of distributing the vaccines to participating vendors. The cost of this program is close to one billion dollars annually as of 1995. Doctors can learn more about this program and how to participate by calling the CDC immunization 800 number (listed in Vaccination Organizations in Resources) and requesting a VCP packet. Children eligible for this program are those without insurance, those underinsured, those eligible for Medicaid, and Native Americans.

The first book reviewed below on the CII, focuses on reducing the non-financial barriers to immunization that the committee responsible for the report felt needed to be addressed along side the financial barriers being overcome by the VCP. The books by Mr. Goldberg and Mr. Grabowski offer a critique of the VCP from a public policy standpoint.

Overcoming Barriers to Immunization
Jane S. Durch, ed. Washington, DC: National Academy Press. 1994. 81 pp. No ISBN. Bibliography.

This book examines strategies for government and private organizations to use for overcoming non-financial barriers to immunization of all under two-year-olds. This book is the report of a workshop held on December 8 and 9, 1993 by the Committee on Overcoming Barriers to Immunization. This eight-member committee was appointed to oversee the workshop by the Division of Health Promotion and Disease Prevention, which is a part of the Institute of Medicine. Committee members, workshop speakers, and participants were mainly from public health and vaccine organizations, and from medical schools, health organizations, and pharmaceutical companies. These included leaders of programs that have tried various approaches to increase immunization rates in their own states or cities. Several pediatricians in private practice also spoke.

The report examines ways to improve the availability of immunizations and increase immunization rates. The committee states that our fragmentary health care system, in which children may be seen by a number of different doctors in different settings, makes it hard to keep track of the immunization status of patients. They cite the 1990 immunization program in Britain, which has a national health care system, as an example of how effective a centrally organized health care system can be in raising immunization rates. They give examples from several states that have linked AFDC (welfare) and WIC services to the immunization status of children. The committee voiced ethical concerns over this practice.

They emphasize the need for health care providers to be better informed and they strongly support the implementation of the CDC's *Standards for Pediatric Immunization Practices* (reviewed in Section E) to help raise immunization levels. In the chapter on building effective communication with families and the community, they state that since some parents are concerned about the safety of vaccines, they recommend providing more information about the risks of the diseases. They also mention parents who object to "unnatural" substances being injected into the body, but they don't elaborate on this point. The overall view they present is that once parents are educated "correctly" they will all want immunizations for their children and if they don't, then incentives, penalties, or legal requirements will make them comply. They support the development of statewide computerized tracking systems to monitor the immunization status of children. The committee cites examples of various private health organizations that have initiated their own immunization programs. For example, the "Every Child by Two" campaign of Betty Bumpers and Rosalyn Carter educates politicians and specifically enlists the services of governors' spouses to spread the message about the need for early immunizations.

In conclusion, the committee hopes that their suggestions will help the nation realize the Childhood Immunization Initiative's goal of a 90% immunization rate of two-year-olds by 1996. The report is footnoted with references from government reports and medical journals.

Available From:
Out of print.

The Search for New Vaccines: The Effects of the Vaccines for Children Program
Henry G. Grabowski. John M. Vernon. Washington, DC: The AEI Press. 1997. 75 pp. ISBN 0-8447-4033-0. Index. Bibliography.

The publisher of this book is a Washington public policy think tank. They also published an earlier book on the Clinton administration's 1993 Vaccines for Children's Program titled, *The Vaccines for Children Program: A Critique*, reviewed in this Section. This book is a follow-up to that book. Both Henry Grabowski and John Vernon are economics professors at Duke University. The authors present an economic analysis of the Vaccines for Children Program (VCP).

The VCP was enacted in 1993 and started on October 1, 1994. It is an entitlement program by which the government pays for vaccines for uninsured and underinsured children. The price that the government pays vaccine manufacturers is negotiated on an annual basis by the CDC. Manufacturers then set their own private price for other purchasers. The government price is much lower than the private price. According to the authors, since the VCP started, the share purchased by the government has increased tremendously, from approximately one-third of U.S. vaccine doses in 1985, to almost two-thirds by 1995. The CDC predicts that the government might eventually buy up as much as 80% of U.S. vaccine doses.

What this means for vaccine manufacturers is the basis of this book. Because the government purchases vaccines at much reduced prices, this large increase in government purchases means a large reduction in profits for vaccine manufacturers. The authors contend that this leaves manufacturers with less money for future research and development (R&D) for new vaccines. While it is true that manufacturers have more funds because of passage of the NVICA in 1986, which freed vaccine makers from lawsuits, changes in government policy that adversely effect their ability to commit money to R&D are felt quickly by them. The authors predict that manufacturers may even shift to making adult vaccines, which are not covered under the VCP, so they can increase profits. However, the authors state that in 1986 there were 285 vaccine R&D projects in progress of which 133 were in clinical trials. Since the authors state that the negative financial effects from the VCP would be most greatly felt on basic research for new vaccines not under development yet, I don't think we have to worry about it anytime soon.

Most of the book is a detailed explanation of how R&D decisions are made and the costs of all phases of vaccine development. I found this quite interesting, so I will relate it here. First, there is a period of basic research and the filing of an investigational new drug (IND) application with the FDA. This is followed by three phases of clinical trials. During phase III clinical trials, the manufacturer files a product license application (PLA) and establishment license application (ELA) with the FDA. The ELA is required only for vaccines among biotechnology products. This means that the FDA must license the manufacturing plant. Approval of the PLA and ELA usually takes two or more years. Once approved, the vaccine can be manufactured. Roughly, four to ten years may pass in development and approval of a new vaccine. One major way vaccine licensure differs from licensure of other biological products, is that phase III clinical trials must use product manufactured in a full-scale commercial plant and not a small pilot facility as is allowed with all other biological and pharmaceutical testing. This means that tens of millions of dollars must be invested in a production plant before the vaccine has even completed its trial period. This makes vaccines a more capital intensive and capital-risky business than other pharmaceutical products, explain the authors.

The authors conclude that because of the extreme high cost and the long number of years necessary to develop a new vaccine, any perceived threat to future revenues will limit the number of future vaccines. Since large government purchases of childhood vaccines through the VCP will reduce profits, the authors see the VCP as unintentionally inhibiting future vaccine development. The authors take their material from government and industry reports.

Available From:
Out of print.

The Vaccines for Children Program: A Critique
AEI Studies in Policy Reform
Robert M. Goldberg, Ph.D. Washington, DC: American Enterprise
Institute Press. 1995. 32 pp. ISBN 0-8447-7052-3. Bibliography.

This may be a slim 32-page booklet, but it packs quite a punch
against the Clinton administration's Vaccines for Children Program
(VCP). Dr. Goldberg is a senior research fellow at the Gordon
Public Policy Center at Brandies University. He has written extensively on health care policy.

The VCP was supported erroneously, Dr. Goldberg contends, by
statistics that claimed that high vaccine costs were preventing poor
children from being immunized. This led to the 1990 measles epidemic the Clinton administration states, because children were not
able to afford the vaccines and overburdened public health clinics
were unable to meet the increased demands for free vaccines. On the
contrary, Dr. Goldberg sites several studies that show that in all but
one or two isolated incidences, all cities involved in the epidemic
had adequate supplies of free vaccines and children had easy access
to them.

The best solution to this supposed lack of access to vaccines and
their high cost, according to the Clinton administration, is federal
purchase and distribution of free vaccines to all uninsured and
underinsured children up to the age of 18. As of 1995, the cost of
this program was near one billion a year and growing rapidly as the
Advisory Committee on Immunization Practices (ACIP), the only
body with control of the VCP, continued to add new free vaccines to
the program.

Dr. Goldberg contends that the statistics supplied by the Clinton
administration claiming that vaccination rates of under two-year-
olds was 55% in 1992 were actually from 1986. 1992 figures were
much higher: 72 – 83% for the six then universal childhood vaccines. Dr. Goldberg believes that vaccine rates are not higher
because parents fail to start their children's vaccinations on time,
that is, at two months of age. A delay in beginning vaccines causes a
delay in receiving all subsequent vaccines. He wants immunization
policies to focus on getting parents to start immunizations at the
recommended age. He also cites the failure of health care staff to
vaccinate when children are seen at clinics for other visits. He even

discusses the experiences of several states and cities that have used various techniques to raise levels, anywhere from a computerized tracking system to issuing a three-month supply of WIC checks if a child's shots are current, instead of just a one-month supply.

Dr. Goldberg concludes very forcefully, that the VCP is a total waste of money, money that could be better spent on other public health programs, for example, by adding funds to Medicaid so states could set up programs as needed to increase immunization rates utilizing various strategies, not just purchasing more vaccines. He states that the VCP was the Clinton administration's "send off" for health care reform, which we all know never passed Congress, and has been used by the Clinton administration as a political tool to show how much the President cares about children's health. Incidentally, after the VCP went into effect on October 1, 1994, the Clinton administration took credit for the large increase in immunization rates of two-year-olds, this time using correct, up-to-date statistics.

This book should interest anyone who wants to understand more about how a health care policy can become part of a political agenda. The book contains footnotes and references from medical sources.

Available From:
American Enterprise Institute Press (8).

Section G.3

Computerized Tracking of Immunization Status

The second half of the 1993 Comprehensive Childhood Immunization Act, otherwise known as the Childhood Immunization Initiative (CII), calling for the implementation of a nation-wide, computerized tracking system to monitor the immunization status of all children did not pass Congress. Instead, the CDC, vaccine advisory groups, and private foundations are actively encouraging states and major cities to develop their own computerized tracking systems.

As of June 2001, the following states have a law authorizing immunization registry: AL, AZ, AR, CA, CO, CT, DE, FL, GA, ID, IN, LA, ME, MD, MI, MS, NH, NY, OR, RI, TN, TX, VA, VT, and WV. Of those states that have a law authorizing immunization registry the following states have required reporting: AZ, AR, CT, DE, GA, ME, MD, MI, MS, TN, TX, VT, and WV. The following states have a law addressing the sharing of immunization information: IA, KS, MN, MO, NE, NC, ND, SD, UT, VA, and WI. There are two types of consent to be in the registry or to share immunization information: required or implied. Except for a handful of states that have not addressed the issue yet, most states have implied consent. The following states have required written consent: HI, ID, IL, IN, KS, LA, MA, NJ, NM, NY, ND, TX, and VA. CA and ND allow verbal consent. Of those who have implied consent, the following states allow one to opt out or limit access: AZ, CT, FL, GA, IA, KY, ME, MD, MI, MN, MT, NE, NH, OH, OK, OR, RI, SD, TN, UT, WA, and WI.

States can receive congressionally mandated funds through the CDC for computer equipment and administration of the registry system. The IOM report *Overcoming Barriers to Immunization* (reviewed in G.2) recommends using computerized tracking systems to provide accurate records of the immunization status of all children, making it easier to keep track of, and notify, children when they need their next shots. It can also eliminate the problem of lost immunization records or the need to take down a child's shot history from multiple doctors, and thus avoid giving a child duplicate shots.

The question of course is how much government interference do we want or need in our task of raising our children? Sending notices to families to remind them to vaccinate their children may be viewed by some as a helpful service and by others as pressure. As long as parents are allowed to voluntarily join the system, it is more likely to be viewed as a helpful service, but if parents are forced or pressured to join, this may less likely be the case.

Section H

The History of Vaccination

It is important to understand how things got the way they are. Therefore, I recommend that you familiarize yourself with the history of vaccination. You will quickly see that it encompasses the study of infectious diseases, bacteriology, virology, cell biology, genetics, microbiology, immunology, as well as many other sub-disciplines. What this all means is that vaccination is not a health issue that can stand on its own, but must be understood in relation to all other biological disciplines. It's just one part of the bigger picture of health and disease.

Below you will find reviews of three books that cover the history of vaccination and two others which highlight particular episodes in that history. Additionally, the book by Stanley Plotkin, *Vaccines*, (reviewed in Section D) also contains extensive histories of the development of vaccines. Unfortunately, all but one of the following books are out of print. Check your local library or request them through interlibrary loan.

A History of Immunization
H. J. Parish, M.D. London: E & S Livingston, Ltd. 1965. 356 pp. Index. Bibliography.

H. J. Parish was formerly Clinical Research Director of Wellcome Research Labs in England. This is a historical account of vaccinations up to 1965. His focus is on the scientists involved in vaccine development. He traces the history of each vaccine individually, dividing each by type of disease (bacterial or viral).

For example, this is the first book where I finally found out the difference between diphtheria toxoid and diphtheria antitoxin. Antitoxin, which was used in the early part of the 20th century, (much of Eleanor McBean's book *The Poisoned Needle* is about this vaccine, see review in Section C) was derived from antibodies created to diphtheria in an animal, usually a horse. Antitoxin provided passive immunity, because you were not actually injected with the disease organism, only the antibodies to it. It tended to have higher adverse reactions than toxoid, mainly due to allergic reactions to the horse protein. Protection against disease "wears off" rather quickly from passive vaccines because the body does not make its own antibodies; it only has "borrowed" antibodies. Diphtheria toxoid, which is used today, is composed of the toxin released by the bacteria that produces the disease. Tetanus toxoid and antitoxin have a similar story.

Because it was published in 1965, this book does not contain information on the newer vaccines, but it is a good resource for explaining the older childhood vaccines and how each was developed.

Available From:
Out of print. Check a medical library.

Magic Shots: A Human and Scientific Account of the Long and Continuing Struggle to Eradicate Infectious Diseases by Vaccination
Allan Chase. NY: William Morrow & Co. 1982. 576 pp.
ISBN 0-688-00787-2. Index. Glossary. Bibliography.

This is a detailed history of vaccination and immunology written for the lay reader. Mr. Chase has spent forty years studying the social and natural history of disease. He has written several other books on health.

Mr. Chase believes vaccines are medicine's greatest weapons against infectious disease. He writes a fascinating history of the development of each of the childhood vaccines. He starts with smallpox vaccine, now no longer in use since the disease has been declared eradicated worldwide. He tells the story of how the germ theory of disease came about. He also has a chapter on the influenza pandemic of 1918-19 . Mr. Chase describes historical vaccine mishaps, but this is viewed as part of the learning process in the development of safer vaccines.

The book is footnoted, mostly with medical sources. It is out of print, but well worth looking for at your local library. It presents a detailed, in-depth examination of the history of immunization.

Available From:
Out of print. Try your local library.

Patenting the Sun: Polio and the Salk Vaccine
Jane S. Smith. NY: Anchor Press. 1991. 413 pp. ISBN 0-385-41868-X.
Index. Bibliography.

Jane Smith was a Polio Pioneer in 1954, which means she participated in the Salk vaccine trails on school children. She writes about this experience and about that generation of children in this book. She holds a Ph.D. and is a writer.

Ms. Smith writes about the baby boom children of the 1950's and how the Salk vaccine trials are a part of their lives and a turning point in the history of the fight against viral diseases. She discusses the March of Dimes at length, at that time called the National Foundation for Infantile Paralysis, and the movers and shakers who researched and promoted the development of the Salk vaccine. She also mentions the Sabin oral polio vaccine.

It is easy reading and is strongly supportive of the Salk vaccine as a lifesaver against the horrors of paralysis and iron lungs. This book is of primary interest for its discussion of the political machinery behind the race for a polio vaccine.

Available From:
Out of print. Try your local library.

Vaccines: Preventing Disease
Michael C. Burge and Don Nardo. San Diego, CA: Lucent Books. 1992.
96 pp. ISBN 1-56006-223-1. Bibliography.

This book is a history of vaccination written for junior high school age children. Both Michael Burge and Don Nardo are writers. Don Nardo specializes in writing non-fiction children's books.

With the use of many illustrations and photographs, the authors describe the basic history of vaccination starting with the Chinese and smallpox back in the middle ages and proceeding onward to tell the story of Edward Jenner, Louis Pasteur, and the polio vaccine trials of the 1950's. The last chapter describes the new vaccines to come: genetically engineered subunit vaccines.

What I found unbelievable to find in a children's book: the development of a contraceptive vaccine is included (!). The authors state that one of the two vaccines now being developed works after fertilization occurs by preventing the embryo from implanting in the uterus. Some may consider this abortion, they state, and thus this particular vaccine may have trouble being accepted. That's an understatement. Why of all the vaccines currently under development, they chose that particular one to include in this book is a sad commentary on our society.

This book is not documented, but the authors include a bibliography of referenced works.

Available From:
Out of print.

A Virus of Love and Other Tales of Medical Detection
Charles T. Gregg. NY: Charles Scribner's Sons. 1983. 310 pp.
ISBN 0-684-17766-8. Index. Bibliography.

Charles Gregg is a biochemist. He devotes two chapters in this book to what he calls the "Swine Flu Caper of 1976". He goes behind the scenes and examines the political maneuvering which led President Gerald Ford to set aside $135 million for mass vaccination of all men, women, and children before the winter of 1976-77 in anticipation of a large and deadly flu epidemic.

It is interesting to note that the campaign almost did not get off the ground because the insurance companies for the vaccine manufacturers refused to insure the vaccines, as they were afraid of a flood of lawsuits due to adverse reactions. Therefore, the government was forced to take financial responsibility for any injuries or deaths caused by the campaign.

Mr. Gregg is a strong supporter of vaccination. He blames the government medical advisors for grossly exaggerating the likelihood of an epidemic and bungling the handling of the situation, thus giving vaccination a bad name.

These two chapters are only 60 pages long and are great reading if you want to see how the political vaccination machine has operated in the past.

Available From:
Out of print. Try your local library.

Section I

Homeopathy and Vaccination

Homeopathy is a system of medicine developed by Dr. Samuel Hahnemann, a German physician, who lived from 1755 to 1843. A homeopathic doctor prescribes homeopathic medicines that would produce in a healthy person the same symptoms that the sick person has. This is based on the idea "like cures like". Homeopathic remedies are very weak biological preparations. The theory is the weaker the dosage the stronger the medicine. To learn more about the theories of homeopathy contact Homeopathic Educational Services or the National Center for Homeopathy listed under Health Organizations in Resources).

Most homeopaths, in accordance with traditional homeopathy, only prescribe these remedies if the person has been exposed to a disease or has actually contracted a disease. This is because treatment is supposed to be individualized and specific for the symptoms. Some homeopaths use homeopathic remedies the same way as vaccines: they administer them to the child in a series of doses before the child is exposed to the disease. This prophylactic use is considered controversial among homeopathic doctors. (Dr. Neustaedter in his book, *The Vaccine Guide*, reviewed in Section A.1, includes a whole chapter on this subject).

A Handbook of Homeopathic Alternatives to Immunisation
Susan Curtis, RSHom. London: Winter Press. 1994. 85 pp.
ISBN 1-874581-02-9. Index. Resources.

Susan Curtis is a homeopathic practitioner living in London. Dr. Curtis briefly discusses her opposition to vaccinations citing short and long-term adverse reactions, but the bulk of the book is devoted to describing various infectious diseases and homeopathic remedies for prevention and treatment.

This book has a two-fold purpose. First, it can be used by travelers who do not wish to receive vaccinations, but nonetheless, may come in contact with infectious diseases which they do not want to contract. She lists the major diseases one may encounter in foreign countries and gives suggestions for homeopathic treatments as both prevention and as remedies. Secondly, the book can be used by parents who do not wish to vaccinate their children, but are interested in homeopathic medicines to prevent the disease or remedies to treat the disease if contracted.

Dr. Curtis includes a *materia medica*, that is, a list of homeopathic medicines, she recommends in the first half of the book. Also included is her suggested first aid kit for travelers and the home. This book is imported from Great Britain so many of the resources she lists are located there.

Available From:
Homeopathic Educational Services (2). The Minimum Price Homeopathic Books (8).

Homeopathy and Immunization
Leslie J. Speight. Essex, England: Health Science Press. 1987. 14 pp. ISBN 0-85032-199-9.

Leslie Speight writes from England. It does not say if he is a doctor. He provides dosage information on different homeopathic medicines to take if your child has been exposed to an immunizable childhood disease. Mr. Speight states that these "vaccines" help bolster the immune system, but immunity conferred by these vaccine will last only about three or four weeks. Therefore, they should be repeated if the child is once again exposed to that particular disease.

It should be noted that both Mr. Speight and Ms. Muir Stanley, in her book reviewed later in this Section, list the same homeopathic vaccines and doses for each disease.

Available From:
The Minimum Price Homeopathic Books (8).

Vaccination? A Review of Risks and Alternatives
Isaac Golden. Canberra, Australia: National Library. 1994. 5th Edition.
85 pp. ISBN 0-7316-8099-5. Footnotes. Resources.

This book is the most detailed one available that explains the use of homeopathic remedies for prevention, as opposed to remedies used after exposure to a disease or once a disease is contracted. Dr. Golden is a naturopathic and homeopathic doctor living in Australia. He is probably the most vocal proponent of homeopathic prophylaxis, especially for use against childhood infectious diseases.

In the first half of the book, he explains why he is opposed to traditional vaccines. He presents graphs showing that disease incidences were on the decline in the UK, Australia, and the U.S. prior to vaccination, although the introduction of vaccination did hasten the decline.

He examines short-term and long-term adverse reactions to vaccines with particular emphasis on the pertussis vaccine. He uses tables that clearly illustrate these adverse reactions. He goes over each childhood vaccine separately. He explains what is contained in the vaccine, describes the disease and gives statistics on vaccine effectiveness.

The second half of the book is devoted to explaining his alternative to traditional (allopathic) vaccines: homeopathic prophylaxis. Dr. Golden has created what he calls a "homeopathic prophylactic kit". This kit contains a series of homeopathic nosodes to be administered at set monthly intervals as "vaccines" against catching the standard immunizable childhood diseases. Nosodes contain actual diseased substances. For example, the nosode, *Pertussin*, contains extremely minute quantities of mucus coughed out from a patient with whooping cough. Dr. Golden is a strong supporter of homeopathic prophylaxis and explains in detail his program of treatment in this book. He also spends around fifteen pages defending his practices against other homeopaths (who are skeptical of this practice) and doctors, as well as government authorities in Australia.

Dr. Golden includes a table which gives suggested homeopathic remedies if your child is exposed to one of these diseases. However, Susan Curtis in her book, *A Handbook of Homeopathic Alternatives to Immunisation*, also reviewed in this Section, provides more detail on treating a disease once it is caught, as does Dr. Starre in his book,

Vaccine Free Prevention and Treatment with Homeopathy, reviewed here, too.

Dr. Golden even mentions God! How wonderful. If health therapies assist the body to cooperate with Natural Law — laws created by God — then, says Dr. Golden, health will result, but if health therapies work against Natural Law (e.g., certain pharmaceutical medicines) then healing is slowed down or stopped.

Dr. Golden's book is well footnoted with medical journal articles and other general vaccination books (e.g., books by Harris Coulter and Viera Scheibner both reviewed elsewhere in this Guide). His use of tables clarifies all his data. Given the controversial nature of homeopathic prophylaxis among homeopaths, the reader may wish to consult with a homeopathic doctor for the latest information on this subject.

Available From:
Homeopathic Educational Services (2). The Minimum Price Homeopathic Books (8).

Vaccinations and Homeopathic Treatment
Heather Muir Stanley. Wantagh, NY: Wholistic Practices, Inc. 1993.
70 pp. No ISBN.

This is a rambling personal essay against vaccination. Ms. Muir Stanley is a long time advocate of natural healing methods and runs a health clinic in Colorado.

After condemning vaccination as harmful to the body and quoting other doctors about possible long-term ill effects, Ms. Muir Stanley describes the current childhood diseases and gives the appropriate homeopathic remedy with dosage instructions. These are to be administered if your child has been exposed to that particular disease. She states that any immunity acquired from using a homeopathic remedy this way is short-lived.

Ms. Muir Stanley briefly discusses the theory behind homeopathy and condemns the disease-oriented medical system that we have in favor of a health-oriented medical system.

This booklet suffers from lack of any chapter breaks or headings of any kind. Nothing is footnoted, though she includes an incomplete bibliography of sources (incomplete, because many of the books do not include the date published or the publisher).

Available From:
Wholistic Practices, Inc. (8).

Vaccine Free Prevention and Treatment with Homeopathy: Alternatives for Domestic and Foreign Disease
Jeffrey J. Starre, MD. Jewel, OH: Two Hearts Medical Publishing. 2000. 95 pp.

This book presents homeopathic remedies for prevention and treatment of common childhood illnesses and tropical diseases. Dr. Jeffrey Starre is a homeopathic physician practicing in Ohio. Dr. Starre wrote this book to answer frequent questions posed by his patients such as, are there safe and effective alternatives to vaccines? Yes, there are he states. His answer is this book.

Since most people are unfamiliar with how homeopathic treatments work, Dr. Starre explains the history of homeopathy and its two basic principles, "like cures like" and "minimum dose, or weakest dose, is more effective". I've only read a little about homeopathy and was always puzzled by the theory that the weaker, or more dilute, the solution the stronger its effect. Dr. Starre includes recent research from physicists who have discovered that at high dilutions, when the substance is no longer physically present, the solution contains a crystalline pattern that is more pronounced the weaker the solution becomes. Somehow, this pattern, which varies from substance to substance, may be responsible for the strong healing powers of the highly diluted preparations. This appears to vindicate homeopaths when critics have argued that "nothing is there".

After this introduction, Dr. Starre describes each of the common "vaccine-preventable" diseases, as well as ones that may be encountered when traveling abroad. For each disease, he describes symptoms and gives a homeopathic remedy suited for those exposed or possibly exposed to the disease. He also gives remedies for those with symptoms and explains how to treat the illness. He includes some patient stories, mainly from his Amish patients, and how the homeopathic remedies were effective in healing them. It should be noted that Dr. Starre does not discuss using homeopathic remedies as "vaccines" for when disease exposure has not occurred or is not likely to occur in the near future.

Dr. Starre advises readers to seek the guidance of a homeopathic physician for treatment, since each of us may respond differently to each remedy. However, for those who can not find a homeopathic doctor (I know they're few and far between here in the Midwest) his instructions are clear enough for readers to use on their own.

Dr. Starre has a Christian perspective and is staunchly pro-life. He indicates in his descriptions of the various vaccines, which ones are grown in aborted fetal tissue or derived from aborted fetuses. He also gives a summary of his major misgivings about vaccines, which includes his concerns that informed choice does not exist because of mandatory laws, and long-term safety has not been tested by controlled studies. Dr. Starre believes that "vaccines are a human experiment with our health being the object of an uncontrolled study".

This book is extremely helpful for parents who are searching for a safer way to prevent and treat disease in their children, instead of using vaccines and pharmaceutical medicines.

Available From:
Out of print. Contact Dr. Jeffrey Starre (8) to see if he may be issuing a reprint.

Section J

International Travel

Whether or not you have vaccinated your children against the routine childhood diseases, if you plan on traveling abroad you may be faced with this decision again. It depends on where you are traveling. Vaccines may be recommended for travel in certain countries or certain areas within a country because the risk of coming in contact with that disease is high.

Only one vaccine is mandatory for travel to certain countries: yellow fever. This is because these countries want to keep yellow fever out of their country. Yellow fever is a viral disease transmitted by mosquito and found in subtropical and tropical areas. You will need an International Certificate of Vaccination (see International Travel in Resources to obtain one) confirming that you have received this vaccine to travel to countries or portions of countries requiring this vaccine. You may have the option to remain in quarantine if you refuse this vaccine, or you may be forced to be vaccinated, or denied entrance to that country.

No vaccines are required to reenter the U.S.

It is in your best interest to inform yourself about the health situation in the areas where you plan to travel. You may have to be quarantined if you are not vaccinated against certain diseases and you are returning from travel in infected areas. According to WHO, quarantinable diseases are yellow fever, cholera, and plague.

If you are interested in homeopathic remedies for these diseases, you may want to read *A Handbook of Homeopathic Alternatives to Immunisation*, reviewed in Section I.

Organizations that can provide you with up-to-the-minute information on health conditions worldwide are listed under International Travel in Resources.

Health Information for International Travel 1999 - 2000

Centers for Disease Control. Washington, DC: Int'l Medical Publishing.
215 pp. ISBN 188320576-X. Index. Glossary.

This book is updated annually by the Centers for Disease Control
(CDC) and provides basic information on immunization requirements and recommendations for foreign travel.

Yellow-colored pages list every country and any required
immunizations. The only required vaccine is yellow fever. It may be
required for two reasons: for anyone entering a specific country, or
for anyone entering a specific country after traveling from a yellow
fever infected country or area.

Also listed is the status of malaria infection in every country.
Detailed information is provided on avoiding malaria.

Another section lists all the diseases for which vaccines are
available. The universal childhood vaccines are included, too. This
section explains who should and should not receive a vaccine, how
effective or safe it is, etc.

If you are planning travel only in developed countries or will be
staying only in tourist areas, vaccines are rarely recommended.
However, if you are going to tropical areas, especially rural areas,
you would be wise to take precautions to avoid disease contact,
whether or not you decide to vaccinate.

Available From:

CDC International Travelers Information Line (7).

Travel and Routine Immunizations: A Practical Guide for the Medical Office, 1998 Edition

Richard F. Thompson, M.D. Milwaukee, WI: Shoreland, Inc. 1998.
229 pp. Index. Bibliography.

Every year since 1991, Dr. Thompson has issued this guide. It is a
comprehensive resource for health care professionals who provide
immunization services, especially to people planning on traveling
abroad. Dr. Thompson is the director of the Occupational Medicine
Services and International Travel Clinic at Camino Medical Group
in Sunnyvale, CA. Dr. Thompson's goal for this book is to provide

health care professionals with the most current and accurate information available on immunizations for almost any circumstances. He updates the book annually and includes a page listing the main changes for that year.

Separate sections cover routine childhood immunizations and special immunizations for international travel. For each vaccine, he briefly describes the disease, the vaccine, who should or should not receive it, side effects, precautions and contraindications, and any special considerations. If different authorities do not agree on a certain item, for example, the manufacturer's product insert may differ from the CDC's recommendation, he notes this. There is also supplemental material covering vaccine storage and handling, record keeping, reporting adverse events, and sample immunization exemption letters for cholera and yellow fever.

A very useful feature is a box at the beginning of each vaccine listing containing "What's New" if anything has changed regarding that vaccine since the previous edition. This makes it easy for the health care provider to keep up-to-date. As Dr. Thompson notes in the introduction, with the increase in the number of new vaccines available in the 1990's, it is more difficult for health care providers to keep abreast of all the recommendations, contraindications, schedules, etc. This book helps to simplify that task. A bibliography contains health authority documents (AAP, CDC, NIP, and WHO) that he consulted in writing this book.

This is a thorough, easy-to-use guide for the immunization provider, especially for those who give vaccines for international travel.

Available From:
Shoreland, Inc. (8).

Section K

Vaccination Programs Around the World

The World Health Organization (WHO) started the Expanded Programme on Immunization (EPI) in 1974 to distribute vaccines for six diseases to developing countries. The vaccines are DPT, polio, measles, and BCG (tuberculosis). The Children's Vaccine Initiative (CVI) was launched in 1990 to help find a "magic bullet", one-dose, multiple antigen vaccine. The CVI has now been made part of the WHO's vaccine programs. The WHO has combined all of its vaccine programs under the umbrella title Global Alliance for Vaccines and Immunization. One of the programs, the Global Fund for Children's Vaccines, was generously funded by the Bill and Melinda Gates Foundation in 1999.

You might be wondering why I include books on third world vaccination campaigns in a guide directed primarily toward U.S. residents. Reading these books raises a lot of important questions about vaccination policies. For example, in developing countries where a much higher number of people die from infectious diseases than in developed countries, do the benefits of vaccines out weigh the risks? Since we have a low rate of "vaccine-preventable" diseases here in the U.S., should we do away with mandatory vaccinations or will disease rates soar as medical authorities fear? Should the ability to pay a high price for a new vaccine be the most important determining factor for its development? If we look at other country's experiences with vaccine programs we may be better able to determine what course of action is best for the U.S.

A Chance to Live: The Heroic Story of the Global Campaign to Immunize the World's Children

Dr. June Goodfield. NY: Macmillan Publishing Co. 1991. 241 pp.
ISBN 0-02-544655-X. Index.

This book is the story of the idea conceived in 1974 by members of the World Health Organization (WHO), UNICEF, the CDC, and other health organizations to vaccinate all the world's children against six childhood infectious diseases by the year 1990. These diseases were polio, measles, diphtheria, pertussis, tetanus, and tuberculosis. June Goodfield is the president of International Health and Biomedics in England and has written several books on medicine and science.

Dr. Goodfield agrees that improved sanitary conditions, more food, better health care, and less crowded conditions would prevent children from getting infectious diseases in developing countries. However, she states that this is a daunting, expensive task beyond the scope of the western world's control. So, the cheaper and more feasible alternative is to send western doctors and nurses to train the local ones and inoculate all children in hopes of preventing some deaths. The original 1990 goal was amended to an 80% vaccination rate and a 90% vaccination rate by the year 2000.

The program is called the Expanded Programme on Immunization (EPI) and is operated by WHO. Dr. Goodfield traveled to many of the targeted countries and describes how the campaign actually took place. She details the obstacles that had to be overcome: language and cultural barriers, wares, government red tape, religious differences, etc. The countries she visited are Turkey, Lebanon, Brazil, and Uganda. The story of the campaign in Uganda takes on a different twist because of the AIDS epidemic there. The big question was whether children with the HIV virus should be vaccinated at all.

At the end of the book, Dr. Goodfield looks to the future and also takes a look at the U.S. She strongly supports vaccination here in the U.S. as vital to insuring our children's health.

Available From:
Out of print. Try your local library.

The Children's Vaccine Initiative: Achieving the Vision
The Committee on the Children's Vaccine Initiative of the Institute of
Medicine. Washington, DC: National Academy Press. 1993. 221 pp.
ISBN 0-309-04940-7. References.

The Children's Vaccine Initiative (CVI) was launched at the World
Summit for Children held in New York City in September 1990.
The purpose of the CVI is to use new technologies to create more
and better vaccines for the world's children. The founders of the
CVI are the Rockefeller Foundation, the UN Development Program,
UNICEF, the World Bank, and WHO. This book is the report of a
committee established by the Institute of Medicine (IOM) which
was asked by U.S. government agencies to formulate a U.S.
response to the CVI, to show how best the U.S. could participate in
the goals of the CVI. The 18-member IOM committee met five
times during the year 1992.

The committee's findings basically are that only the four commercial vaccine manufacturers in the U.S. are of a large enough size
and have the finances to help develop the numerous new vaccines
wanted by the CVI. The ideal CVI vaccine, or "super vaccine", is a
one-dose vaccine containing multiple antigens to many diseases,
given orally shortly after birth, heat stable, and affordable. Until
such an ideal vaccine can be made, the CVI is working to produce
other vaccines using the technology of genetic engineering. Since
markets in developing countries can afford to pay little for vaccines,
it has not been financially feasible for U.S. manufacturers to invest
in developing vaccines that are to be used solely in other countries.
Noting the fragmentary structure behind vaccine research, development, and use, the IOM committee suggested the establishment of a
U.S. government agency (e.g., a National Vaccine Authority
(NVA)), which would help with federal funding of research and
development of the needed new vaccines, help absorb legal liabili-
ties, and guarantee markets for the vaccines.

Also discussed are the political and legal aspects of vaccine
development and explanations of how vaccine technology should be
used in the U.S. to help other countries, as well as develop new and
safer vaccines for use in the U.S.

The book contains a few footnotes, but this is not a scholarly
research book. It is a report of a committee's findings and it

therefore is only a summary of information and a recommendation for future U.S. course of action.

Available From:
National Academy Press (8).

Every Second Child
Archie Kalokerinos, M.D. Melbourne, Australia: Thomas Nelson and Sons. 1974. 200 pp. Index. Bibliography.

Archie Kalokerinos is a doctor who worked among the Aborigines of Australia beginning in 1957. He was concerned with the extremely high infant mortality rate, which in some areas was as high as 500 in 1000, hence, the name of this book. After ten years of serving these people and endless research, he made a breakthrough in 1967: the infants were suffering from a Vitamin C deficiency that led them to be easily susceptible to disease. He spent many more years convincing the medical authorities of his findings. His struggles are related in this fascinating book.

And what does this have to do with vaccinations? In the early 1970's when a mass vaccination campaign was started among a particular group of Aborigines, Dr. Kalokerinos found that the infant mortality rate doubled from deaths due to other illnesses. He finally concluded that the vaccinations were destroying the Vitamin C stores in the body, which in these infants were already low, and this made the babies even more susceptible to disease. Dr. Kalokerinos does not make clear which vaccinations he is referring to. Do all vaccines or only certain ones have this draining effect on Vitamin C stores in the body? In other books, I have read that measles drains Vitamin C stores, so perhaps measles vaccine has this same effect. At times, Dr. Kalokerinos mentions tetanus and diphtheria vaccines; otherwise he does not specify particular vaccines.

At the time he wrote this book, Dr. Kalokerinos did not oppose vaccination. He was just very concerned that care be taken in their administration. However, since then he has become an outspoken critic of vaccination.

Available From:
Global Vaccine Awareness League (1). New Atlantean Press (8).

Legitimate Immunity versus Medical Chaos: Transcending the Futile Dream of Universal Immunization
Raymond Obomsawin. Quebec, Canada: Canadian Natural Health Society. 1992. 160 pp. No ISBN. Typed report. Footnotes. Bibliography.

This is a report on the current status of Canada's International Immunization Program (CIIP). It does not state in the report who Raymond Obomsawin is, however, he does relate in the introduction that he visited northeast Thailand in March 1990 to carry out a field evaluation of the WHO Expanded Programme on Immunization (EPI) initiative there. He shares his observations and conclusions in this report.

Mr. Obomsawin states that he is presenting a one-sided (i.e., negative) view of immunization to counter-balance the almost 100% positive government immunization reports. He is concerned that the EPI has not helped stop the spread of disease and that immunizations possibly weaken children's immune systems so they more easily succumb to other diseases. He fully documents his theories with government reports and first-hand accounts.

He also briefly presents the history of immunization and its role in stopping the spread of infectious disease. He includes numerous graphs showing that infectious disease was declining before the introduction of immunizations. Some graphs are for third world countries and show a rise in cases after mass immunization programs were started. He lists short and long-term adverse reactions. He discusses immune system malfunction. Unfortunately, when he leaves the topic of immunization programs in the third world, he stops using government reports and medical journals as source materials and relies heavily on alternative health books and magazines, and other general works opposing vaccinations (in particular, books by Randall Neustaedter, Cynthia Cournoyer and Walene James — all reviewed in other Sections) as source material.

He suggests a different approach to ensuring the health of children (and adults) in developing countries: focus on the health of the soil and better nutrition. He explains the link between nutrients, soil, farming techniques, and agri-chemicals on our health.

It's written in a "government report" style consisting of dry language and long, convoluted sentences. Everything is thoroughly footnoted. It's must reading for anyone seriously interested in the possible negative impact of immunization campaigns on developing countries.

Available From:
Canadian Natural Health Society (2).

The Politics of International Health: The Children's Vaccine Initiative and the Struggle to Develop Vaccines for the Third World
William Muraskin. Albany, NY: State University of New York Press. 1998. 258 pp. ISBN 0-7914-4000-1. Index. Bibliography.

This fascinating and readable book is the story of the men and women involved in the founding and development of the Children's Vaccine Initiative (CVI) and their struggle to achieve their goal of creating a perfect "children's vaccine". Mr. Muraskin is Professor of Urban Studies at Queens College, City University of New York. Mr. Muraskin takes what some might consider a dull, heavy topic, and turns it into an exciting story by filling his book with the thoughts and words of the actual people involved in the CVI, many of whom he personally interviewed.

The CVI was announced at the time of the World Summit on Children in New York City in September 1990. (I was living in New York City then and I remember all the attention this summit received). Mr. Muraskin explains how the CVI came to be and what its goals were. He states that getting needed vaccines to the third world was a difficult task because of the great fragmentation between all the groups responsible for basic research, applied research, product and development, and product delivery. The 1970's and 1980's saw a move away from public sector control of vaccine manufacturing and development, and a subsequent shift to a few private pharmaceutical companies making most of the vaccines, especially here in the U.S. He states that during the 1980's, pharmaceutical companies "woke up" to the possibility of making large profits from vaccines and started raising their prices to third world countries. At this time, the Expanded Programme on Immunization (EPI) of WHO was the largest international organization involved in vaccine delivery to developing countries.

The scientists who founded the CVI saw the need for an organization to bring together the following three parts of the vaccine process: (1) basic research on new vaccines, which was mainly scientist-initiated and independent of eventual need or product use; (2) product development people, i.e., the pharmaceutical companies who took the basic research and developed and tested and actually produced a new vaccine with a cost of from anywhere between 50 – 200 million dollars; and (3) the people out in the field who desperately wanted vaccines that would work better in tropical countries with fewer side effects and fewer doses. All of these groups, Mr. Muraskin states oddly enough, worked in isolation from each other.

The CVI had an even bigger agenda than just coordinating the work of these various groups. They wanted to develop the "children's vaccine": a one shot "magic bullet" that would contain antigens from a multitude of diseases, never need a booster, had no side effects, and was heat stable (that is, not needing constant refrigeration, something that was difficult to maintain in remote tropical areas). This grandiose goal served to get the CVI started, but it has remained elusive.

The CVI's original goal was to work on product development, which was solely in the hands of the private sector, and coordinate this with researchers and those in the field. The CVI needed the cooperation of vaccine manufacturers, because countries only give pharmaceutical product licenses to the actual manufacturer and the CVI was not in the business of actually manufacturing vaccines. The CVI found it very difficult to interest private companies in improving vaccines for use in the developing world when there was no market for them in developed countries. For example, the CVI originally supported the development of a more heat-stable polio vaccine. It took them time, but they were able to convince two vaccine manufacturers to produce the vaccine although there was no need for it in developed countries. The vaccine didn't get produced however, because of internal conflicts between the CVI and the EPI.

Mr. Muraskin explains how difficult it was for the CVI to work in the waters of the international health agencies that, who did not like their "turf" being stepped on. He describes in detail the trouble with the WHO and distrust among the Europeans and Americans, as well as personality clashes among the CVI founders. In the end, the CVI failed to remain an independent organization and is now under the wing of WHO.

Mr. Muraskin is a strong supporter of vaccination and the right of third world children to receive better vaccines. He is not afraid to detail the personality conflicts, pride, and prejudices among the players in the international vaccine scene, especially when he believes that their actions have jeopardized their goals. Because Mr. Muraskin shows the individuals at work in the CVI, the book is fascinating. You are made to realize how much impact one person or just a handful of individuals can have upon the world. The book is footnoted and referenced with letters, personal interviews, and government documents. This is a fascinating look at the politics of international vaccination campaigns.

Available From:
SUNY Press (8).

Vaccines and World Health: Science, Policy and Practice
Paul F. Basch. NY: Oxford University Press. 1994. 274 pp.
ISBN 0-19-508532-9. Bibliography. Index.

This book describes ways to increase vaccine acceptance by developing countries and the placement of infrastructures to make vaccines available to those most in need. It is not technical and serves as an interesting description of worldwide vaccine policies. The author, Mr. Basch, writes from Stanford, CA. It is not stated anywhere, but I assume that he is a professor there. Mr. Basch believes that vaccines are a major part of preventive health care, especially in disease-ridden areas of the world.

Mr. Basch begins by discussing the ups and downs of "technology transfer", that is, the movement of technology from concept to actual use. He emphasizes the problems of placing and using western technology in developing countries. He quickly focuses on health care technologies and the special programs promoting the use of vaccines. He devotes an entire chapter to explaining the need for regulation of technology policies by government bodies, for example, how health technology should be funded, produced, marketed, etc. He then applies this to specific cases of government regulation in developing countries that ensure adequate vaccines for their populations.

Several sections are noteworthy. Mr. Basch explains the cultural context of health and lists various "misconceptions" held by villagers, which keeps them from getting their children vaccinated. For instance, one is that "immunizations will keep you from never getting sick again". Okay, we know that's not true, but others are more borderline. For example, "sick children should not be immunized" is considered a misconception. He notes also that even doctors in the U.S. may hold this erroneous view. This seems to come from the recent push here in the U.S. to allow as few contraindications as possible.

One whole chapter is devoted to describing "The Global Vaccine Establishment" and explaining the various world health agencies and programs and what their role is in promoting vaccination. This should be of interest to anyone wanting to learn more about the infrastructure of worldwide vaccination campaigns.

Several appendices introduce the technology behind the development of new generation vaccines and how they utilize recent breakthroughs in genetic engineering.

This book is quite fascinating. Mr. Basch has done a tremendous amount of research and everything is documented, mostly from medical journals. Anyone interested in learning about the worldwide scope of vaccine distribution and use should read this book.

Available From:
Oxford University Press (8).

RESOURCES

Resources

Introduction

The organizations and companies included here can provide you with a wealth of information on vaccinations and other health topics. I have divided the resources by type of organization, e.g., vaccine organizations, health organizations, publishers, etc. Listings are alphabetical within each group. Organizations that are primarily involved with legal exemptions to vaccinations are listed under Legal Exemptions. Ones that are primarily health organizations, but who have an interest in vaccines are listed under Health Organizations. The Vaccine Injuries section contains contact information for submitting claims to the NVICP and reports to VAERS. Under Pediatric Vaccines you will find listed all of the universally recommended childhood vaccines in the U.S. along with a summary of vaccine ingredients and vaccine manufacturers' addresses.

If you contact these organizations by mail, please consider enclosing a SASE with your request. Many of these groups operate on a shoestring budget and postage costs add up quickly. They will appreciate your thoughtfulness.

Each of the resource sections is numbered and these numbers correspond to the numbers in parentheses found under "Available From" in the book reviews. Book titles, authors, names, and current prices are indicated. The letter in parentheses following the book price refers to the section in the book reviews where the review of that book appears. For example "*A Shot in the Dark*, H. Coulter, $10.95 (B.2)" means that this book is reviewed in Section B, subsection 2. All prices listed are for paperbacks unless noted as hardcover by "hc".

Do not neglect to check your local library for these books. You may be able to obtain them through interlibrary loan. Medical textbooks, which usually have high price tags, can be found in medical school libraries or you can request them through interlibrary loan. Your research need not be expensive.

Some of these books are published by small presses or self-published and not readily available in bookstores or libraries. Where this is the case, I have attempted to list every source that I could find that sells that book. I have included the large publishers too, but you should be able to easily find their books in a bookstore, or order them through a bookstore. You can find many of these books, from small or large publishers, at online bookstores such as Amazon.com or Barnes and Noble (bn.com).

Some organizations sell so many vaccination books that the complete list is cumbersome to include. In that case, I mention this in the listing and encourage you to send for their complete book list or catalog. However, I do list these organizations under "Available From" in the book reviews, so you can tell if they currently carry that book.

Information changes rapidly. To find out about changes between editions, visit our website at http://www.patterpublications.com. Here you can find updates to the resources.

Diane Rozario

1

Vaccination Organizations

You will find a variety of vaccine organizations from the U.S. and Canada listed here, ranging from government funded research organizations, to parent-initiated information groups. Some are staunchly pro-vaccine, some are firmly anti-vaccine, while others are all shades in between. Some are only local or state-wide groups, others are national or international in scope.

Arizona Vaccine Information Network
Kelly Larsen
602-978-6804
email: midwife1@uswest.net
http://www.azavenue.com/kelly/organizations.htm

Their website contains a vast listing of vaccine-related internet resources.

The Association for Vaccine Damaged Children (AVDC)
67 Shier Dr.
Winnipeg, Manitoba R3R 2H2 Canada
204-895-9192
email: tjames@autobahn.mb.ca

This association is organizing a class action lawsuit that will include many vaccine-damaged children. If they are successful, this will lend additional credibility when discussing the issue of vaccine informed consent and choice with legislators in Canada.

California Vaccine Awareness
Dawn Winkler, President
970-641-7413
cvainfo@yahoo.com

CVA is a grassroots network of parents and doctors dedicated to promoting informed decisions regarding vaccination and protecting parents' rights to make their own choice. CVA has a free group email list and will be raising funds for much needed research regarding the effects of vaccination. In 2001, CVA successfully stopped the mandating of hepatitis A and PREVNAR vaccines for school entry in California.

Citizens for Healthcare Freedom, Inc.
Alan Phillips, Director
P.O. Box 62282
Durham, NC 27715
email: alan_phillips@unc.edu
http://www.unc.edu/~aphillip/www/vaccine/informed.htm

CHF is a nonprofit corporation providing educational lectures, information and vaccine support to North Carolina residents primarily, and to other citizens internationally. Co-founding director Alan Phillips is the author of "Dispelling Vaccination Myths," an internationally published report. You can view or download this report for free from their website. This report is available along with a resource directory, religious exemption information, and a copy of North Carolina vaccine laws, in their "North Carolina Vaccine Kit" for $12 ppd. CHF is managed by volunteers.

Classen Immunotherapies, Inc.
Dr. J. Bart Classen, MD, MBA
6517 Montrose Ave.
Baltimore, MD 21212
410-377-4549
http://www.vaccines.net

Classen Immunotherapies is a privately owned research stage biopharmaceutical company committed to developing safer vaccines and preventing chronic immune system disorders. Dr. Classen, an immunologist, established it. They are especially concerned about a link between vaccines and the development of diabetes. Their website explains their research and presents information on problems with the safety of current vaccines.

Coalition For Informed Choice (CFIC)
Gary Krasner, Director
188-34 87th Drive, Ste. 4B
Hollis, NY 11423
718-479-2939
email: gk-cfic@juno.com

CFIC assists people seeking to become advocates against vaccination, and to promote personal freedom of choice in decisions about health. They help people organize locally with like-minded people, and provide advice on the nuts and bolts of effective advocacy. All contributions (payable to "CFIC"), go towards the advancement of these goals, and are greatly appreciated. Credited reproductions of CFIC publications or articles by Gary Krasner are permitted.

CFIC provides advice to parents on the correct way to claim the New York State personal religious exemption from childhood vaccinations required for school. For $20 (check payable to "CFIC") parents will receive (via email only) a 100+ page report. It contains important do's and don'ts, and examples of how to deal with the most common objections from school officials. It is general enough for most people's purposes and should be successful in most instances. However, it doesn't cover every possible situation and complication. The report is routinely updated and updates are available free to previous purchasers.

Concerned Parents for Vaccine Safety
Marie Van-Es, President
12709 99th Ct. E
Puyallup, WA 98373
253-445-2514

The goal of this group is to educate parents on the possible dangers
and ineffectiveness of vaccines so they can make an informed decision. They have support group meetings.

Connecticut Vaccine Information Alliance
Lisa F. Reiss
P.O. Box 161
Manchester, CT 06045
860-231-2231
email: info@ctvia.org
http://www.ctvia.org

This group keeps abreast of vaccine information for Connecticut
parents. They publish a newsletter and maintain a website.

The Eagle Foundation, Inc.
154 Provencher Blvd.
Winnipeg, Manitoba R2H 0G3 Canada
email: eaglefoundation@home.com

This is a non-profit organization founded in 1995 by three chiropractors. They help families of vaccine-damaged children and
provide others with assistance and information on vaccine issues.

Global Alliance for Vaccines and Immunization (GAVI)
Lisa Jacobs, GAVI Secretariat
c/o UNICEF
Palais des Nations
1211 Geneva 10, Switzerland
email: gavi@unicef.ch
http://www.vaccinealliance.org

The mission of the GAVI is to fulfill the right of every child throughout the world to be protected against vaccine-preventable diseases of public health concern. To achieve this goal the GAVI is trying to improve access to vaccination services, expand the use of vaccines, and accelerate the development of new vaccines especially for developing countries. To this end, the GAVI has set up the "Global Fund for Children's Vaccines" (see separate listing in this section). The GAVI is composed of a board of twelve members representing its major partners: WHO, UNICEF, the World Bank, the Rockefeller Foundation and vaccine manufacturers.

Global Fund for Children's Vaccines
Bill and Melinda Gates Children's Vaccine Program (CVP)
4 Nickerson St.
Seattle, WA 98109-1699
206-285-3500
206-285-6619
email: info@childrensvaccine.org
http://www.childrensvaccine.org

This fund was started by the GAVI (see listing above). It has been generously funded with seed money from the Bill and Melinda Gates Foundation, who are giving $750 million over a five-year period starting in 1999. The purpose of the fund is to finance under-utilized and new vaccines, increase vaccine access, and improve research and development of priority vaccines for developing countries. It was publicly launched on January 31, 2000. The CVP's aim is to provide equal access to new vaccines for children worldwide. Initially, they are focusing on vaccines for respiratory, diarrheal, and liver disease. Their website contains many educational articles, links to other sites, and details about their activities.

Global Vaccine Awareness League (GVAL)

25422 Trabuco Rd. Ste. 105-230
Lake Forest, CA 92630
949-929-1191
email: michelle@gval.com
http://www.gval.com

GVAL is a non-profit, educational organization founded in 1995 by
Michelle Helms-Gaddie after the vaccine-related death of her 25-
month old son. Dr. Viera Scheibner is the chairperson of their board
of directors. They seek to educate parents about the possible risks of
vaccinations so they can make an informed choice. There are three
types of annual membership: basic - $40; supporting - $65; and
professional - $125. Membership through the internet is also avail-
able at $20 a year. They sell vaccine books by Viera Scheibner
(B.2), Neil Miller (A.1), Robert Mendelsohn (A.2), Grace Girdwain
(F), and copies of state immunization laws and other materials and
tapes. Visit their website to see their book list, or call, or write. A
quarterly newsletter is included with membership.

Health World Online: Vaccination Center

http://www.healthy.net/vaccine

This webpage contains information on vaccines from Randall
Neustaedter, author of *The Vaccine Guide* (A.1). Dr. Neustaedter
also has his own website at http://www.cure-guide.com.

Illinois Vaccine Awareness Coalition (IVAC)

Barbara Alexander Mullarkey, Spokeswoman
P.O. Box 946
Oak Park, IL 60303
847-836-0488

The mission of IVAC is to educate people on vaccine ingredients,
contraindications, adverse reactions, studies, statistics and legal
exemptions for informed vaccine choice. IVAC's goals are to prevent vaccine-related deaths, brain damage, and physical disabilities
due to vaccines. They are currently attempting to get a philosophical

exemption clause added to the state immunization laws. They are also trying to stop the chicken pox vaccine from being added to the list of required childhood vaccines in Illinois. Send a SASE for an information flyer explaining their activities and a publications list. They have the following print material available: "To Vaccinate or Not to Vaccinate?" 90 pp. booklet, $9 + $1.60 p&h. A collection of Ms. Mullarkey's newspaper columns on vaccines from 1988-1994, 24 pp. booklet, $7 + $1.60 p&h. Reprints of IVAC's "Letters to the Editor" from 1998-1999 with pointers on how to get your letters published, 30 pp., $7 + $1.60 p&h. "Illinois Children Caught in the Vaccine Roulette", stories about vaccine-damaged children in Illinois, 15 pp. booklet, $5 +$1.60 p&h. Make checks payable to "NutraVoice".

Immunization Action Coalition (IAC)
Hepatitis B Coalition
1573 Selby Ave., Suite 234
St. Paul, MN 55104
651-647-9009
email: admin@immunize.org
http://www.immunize.org

The IAC is a source for child, adolescent, and adult vaccine information. Their mission is to boost immunization rates. The Hepatitis B Coalition is a program of the IAC specifically promoting hepatitis B vaccination. The IAC provides many free print materials explaining the benefits of immunizations. You can also print out current CDC VIS's, and other CDC documents from their website. Their website contains extensive links to other pro-immunization websites. They have a free email newsletter called "IAC Express". Write or call to request a copy of their catalog listing all their print materials, many free, or visit their website to download many of these materials.

Immunization, Vaccination & You (IVY)
IVY League Foundation
P.O. Box 1007
Rosamond, CA 93560
661-824-1032

Founded in 1999, IVY's primary purpose is to conceive, initiate, conduct, facilitate, investigate, and freely disseminate results of vaccine research in order to improve immunization policies and to insure adequate informed consent and continued protection of parental rights. They emphasize vaccine safety and developing better ways to detect those children who are at high-risk of being injured by vaccines, especially detecting possible genetic predispositions.

Informed Consent Movement
5615 Morningside Dr., Suite 222
Houston, TX 77005-3218

The Informed Consent Movement provides support to those persons seeking information for making informed decisions regarding vaccinations. Members of this movement hold "Vaccination Education" workshops. They also do seminars and have print materials available.

Inoculation Discussion Group of Omaha
Mrs. Carla Mowry
402-455-6339
email: pcrc_mow@ix.netcom.com

They are a source of vaccine information for Nebraska residents. They hold meetings in Omaha.

The Institute for Vaccine Safety (IVS)
Johns Hopkins Bloomberg School of Public Health
Neal A. Halsey, M.D., Director
615 N Wolfe St, Suite 5515
Baltimore, MD 21205-2179
email: info@vaccinesafety.edu
http://www.vaccinesafety.edu

The purpose of the IVS is to provide objective information on the
safety of immunizations. They believe because they are part of an
independent academic institution that they can provide objective and
accurate information on vaccine safety in a timely fashion, unlike
government officials who are slow to provide information because
of restrictions placed on them, legal concerns, or fears of misinter-
pretation of their findings. IVS has established a website to quickly
get information to the public, journalists, vaccine manufacturers,
and government agencies. They are planning to launch a quarterly
newsletter summarizing recent developments in vaccine safety.
They hold seminars and workshops at Johns Hopkins University.

Long Island Vaccination Information Networking Group (L.I.V.I.N.G.)
Anne Attivissimo, President
P. O. Box 432
Centerport, NY 11721
email: LIVING2693@aol.com

L. I. V. I. N. G. is a non-profit organization, which recognizes that
public awareness is the greatest prevention against vaccine injuries
and deaths. They support each individual's right to informed consent. They are a resource center for those who wish to seek information on vaccine issues.

Massachusetts Citizens for Vaccination Choice (MCVC)
Debbie Bermudes, Executive Director
P.O. Box 1033
East Arlington, MA 02474-0020
781-646-4797
email: mcvchq@juno.com
http://www.vaccinechoice.org

MCVC is a non-profit education and advocacy organization composed of parents, professionals, and concerned others from across the state. Some have vaccinated their children completely, others have chosen to decline all vaccinations, while still others have decided to accept certain vaccines but not all. What unites them is their belief that unbiased information should be readily accessible and choice should rest with the individual. Their mission is to provide information and resources to help individuals make informed vaccination decisions.

Michigan Opposing Mandatory Vaccines (MOM)
Suzanne Waltman, President
P.O. Box 1121
Troy, MI 48099-1121
586-447-2418
email: mom@salineguide.com
http://www.salineguide.com/mom

MOM is a non-profit organization that supports the right of parents to make educated choices about vaccines and health care for themselves and their children. To this end they oppose mandatory vaccinations and actively lobby state legislators. They were successful in defeating a state bill in 1995 that would have taken away the philosophical exemption in Michigan. They issue a newsletter containing updates of their activities. Membership is $15 a year and includes the thrice yearly newsletter. You can purchase audio or video tapes of their vaccine conferences, as well as other vaccine books from them.

National Immunization Program (NIP)
NIP Public Inquiries
Mail Stop E-05
1600 Clifton Road NE
Atlanta, GA 30333
800-232-2522 NIP Hotline
888-CDC-FAXX (232-3299) Fax Information Service – toll free
http://www.cdc.gov/nip

The NIP was established in 1993 as a successor to the Division of Immunization within the CDC's National Center for Prevention Services. The NIP administers grants to states to support Immunization Action Plans (IAPs). (IAPs are plans implemented by states and major urban areas to achieve 90% immunization rates of all two-year-olds.) The NIP is also the agency responsible for the operational aspects of the Clinton Administration's Childhood Immunization Initiative (see Section G.2).

There are several ways to get information and materials from the CDC. You can call the NIP Hotline to (1) request the name of a nearby health clinic that administers vaccinations; (2) get answers to commonly asked questions; or (3) request publications. You can download a copy of the "CDC/NIP Resource Request List" from their website. Single copies of NIP materials are free and include many items among them: *Parents Guide to Childhood Immunization* (A.1); Vaccine Information Statements (A.1); *Standards for Pediatric Immunization Practices* (E); *Guide to Contraindications to Childhood Vaccinations* (B.1); and *Epidemiology and Prevention of Vaccine-Preventable Diseases (The Pink Book)* (E). All items are free except *The Pink Book*. You can read it free on their website or purchase a copy by calling the Public Health Foundation at toll free 877-252-1200 ($25 + p&h).

National Network for Immunization Information (NNII)
66 Canal Center Plaza, Suite 600
Alexandria, VA 22314
http://www.idsociety.org (click on the NIIN icon on the IDSA home page)

This organization changed its name in 1999 from the "Vaccine Initiative" to the National Network for Immunization Information. It is a project of the Infectious Disease Society of America (IDSA), the Pediatric Infectious Disease Society (PIDS), the AAP, and the American Nurses Association (ANA). Their aim is to provide scientifically valid vaccine information to the public, health professionals, policy makers, and the media. They wish to be a source for independent vaccine information.

National Vaccine Information Center (NVIC)
421-E Church St.
Vienna, VA 22180
800-909-SHOT
703-938-DPT3
703-938-5768 Fax
email: info@909shot.com
http://www.909shot.com

NVIC is a national, non-profit educational organization founded in 1982 by Barbara Loe Fisher and Kathi Williams that seeks to prevent needless vaccine injuries and deaths. Originally called Dissatisfied Parents Together, they formed to voice their disapproval of the continued use of the whole-cell, killed pertussis vaccine. They have since changed their name and broadened their goals. They were active in lobbying for the National Childhood Vaccine Injury Act passed by Congress in 1986 and have closely monitored the National Vaccine Injury Compensation Program, which this act set up. They pushed for use of the acellular pertussis vaccine in the U.S. They are currently involved in gathering information on short and long-term adverse reactions to various childhood vaccines. They have established their own database of vaccine adverse reaction reports.

Individual membership is $25 a year. Professional membership is $50 a year. Membership includes their newsletter "The Vaccine Reaction". Materials which they publish include: *The Consumer's Guide to Childhood Vaccines*, $9 (A.1); "The Compensation System and How it Works", $5; "Law Firm Directory", $5; Autism-Vaccination Packet, $15 ppd.; Polio Contamination Packet, $16 ppd. Shipping is $4.50 minimum or 10% for book orders. They also sell other books, videos, and, audio tapes. Check their website for a complete listing or write or call for a free publication list.

National Vaccine Program Office
888-246-2675 toll free
email: NVPO@cdc.gov
http://www.cdc.gov/od/nvpo

The NVPO was created by the 1986 NCVIA law. The CDC runs it. It provides leadership and coordination among federal agencies to help implement the goals of the National Vaccine Plan. They deal with DHHS, USDA, DOD, WHO, vaccine manufacturers, consumer groups, and academic institutions. Check their website for information on their activities. You can read the 1994 National Vaccine Plan on their website (reviewed in Section G.1).

New Jersey Alliance for informed Choice in Vaccination
(NJ-AICV)
Dr. Renee Foster, DC, Director
Sue Collins, Assistant Director
PO Box 243
Gillete, NJ 07933
800-613-9925
732-290-9054 fax
email: NJAICV@aol.com

The NJ-AICV is an advocacy group concerned with defending the freedom of all New Jersey citizens to make informed, voluntary, vaccination decisions. Their goal is to protect the right to informed consent through education and awareness.

New Yorkers for Vaccination Information and Choice (NYVIC)
PO Box 287 342
New York, NY 10128
212-473-8201
212-873-5051 (recorded announcement)
email: nyvic@nyvic.org
http://www.nyvic.org

NYVIC, formerly known as the Natural Immunity Information Network, provides information to help parents make an informed choice about vaccinations. They hold monthly support meetings the first

Sunday of each month. You can also post questions on their online forum.

Parents Requesting Open Vaccine Education (PROVE)
Dawn Richardson
P.O. Box 91566
Austin, TX 78709-1566
email: prove@vaccineinfo.net
http://vaccineinfo.net

PROVE provides information on vaccines, and immunization policies and practices that affect the children and adults of Texas. Their mission is to prevent vaccine injury and death and to promote and protect the right of every person to make informed independent vaccination decisions for themselves and their families. Free email vaccine newsletter. Donations accepted.

Pennsylvania Parents for Vaccine Awareness (PPVA)
P.O. Box 173
Mill Village, PA 16427
814-796-4000
814-825-1071
email: ppva@velocity.net

This group in northeast Pennsylvania holds monthly informational meetings for anyone wanting to know more about vaccinations so they can make an informed choice. A minimum donation of $15 a year is suggested for membership.

People Advocating Vaccine Education (PAVE)

Lisa Jillani, Director
P. O. Box 36701
Charlotte, NC 28236
email: WeRPAVE@yahoo.com
http://www.vaccines.bizland.com

PAVE is a group that supports the rights of parents to decide whether or not to vaccinate themselves or their children. They hold meetings every other month to share information on vaccine issues. Introductory membership is $5 a year and includes a bimonthly newsletter. Enclose an SASE for free information on specific questions (or email them).

Utah Vaccine Awareness Coalition

6337 Highland Dr., Suite 135
Salt Lake City, UT 84121
801-243-3526
801-273-0209 fax
email: goffe5@micron.net

This organization keeps abreast of vaccine changes and policies, and educates parents and caregivers about vaccine choices. They sell Robin Goffe's book, *I Don't Want to Be Ty*, for $12.00 + $3.00 p&h. As of Winter 2002, they are reorganizing.

Vaccination and Childhood Disease Discussion Group

Joan Batista
Arlington, MA
email: BatistaJ@aol.com
http://hometown.aol.com/batistaj/myhomepage/index.html

This is a monthly discussion group for parents and parents-to-be. They discuss all aspects of childhood vaccination as well as alternative treatments for some vaccinated-against and other diseases. Their goal is to act as a resource for making informed vaccination decisions. Check the website for meeting information.

Vaccination Risk Awareness Network (VRAN)
P.O. Box 169
Winlaw, BC V0G 2J0
Canada
250-355-2525
email: eddawest@netidea.com
http://www.vran.org

VRAN provides information on the risks of vaccines and helps parents in making informed decisions. They provide support for parents of vaccine-damaged children. Membership is $25 a year and includes their quarterly newsletter. A vaccine information packet is $7.00 + $2.50 p&h Canadian funds.

Vaccine Information and Action in Maryland (VIAM)
Amanda Buxbaum, Director
8632 Garfield Street
Bethesda, MD 20817
301-897-8962
email: viam@earthlink.net
http://www.viam.f2s.com

VIAM was formed in January 2000. They hold monthly informational meetings and several members are available for informational presentations on request. They send out monthly email letters. They advocate for informed consent and parental choice.

Vaccine Information and Awareness (VIA)
Karin Schumacher, President
12799 La Tortola
San Diego, CA 92129
619-339-5498
858-484-1187 fax
email: via@access1.net
http://www.access1.net/via

VIA supports pro-informed choice regarding vaccinations. They seek to educate parents about all sides of the vaccine issue. Their main project is a vast website offering links to many vaccine resources such as, legal issues, diseases, news groups, alternative medicine, pet vaccines, and scores of websites both pro-vaccine and pro-informed choice. They actively support the adding of philosophical exemptions to state immunization laws.

Karin has put together an "immunization information package" that contains vaccine manufacturers' product inserts, a resource list of pro-choice immunization groups, informed consent information sheets, a booklist of over 75 vaccine-related books and publications, an article on starting a grass roots organization, your state vaccine law and a list of states with philosophical exemptions, vaccine current events articles, as well as other items. This package is $20 ppd.

A law article authored by Karin titled "Informed Consent: Should It Be Extended to Vaccination?", published in the Fall 1999 issue of the Thomas Jefferson Law Review, is available for $10 ppd. It explores informed consent from legal and medical perspectives.

Vaccine Network
Christina S. Abel, RN, Director
3411 Winnetka Ave. N
Crystal, MN 55427-2020
email: christinasabel@hotmail.com

This is a Minnesota vaccination organization with information about current childhood disease rates in Minnesota, as well as information on the history of disease outbreaks in that state. They hold meetings several times a year. They have a list of recommended books on vaccinations that are available in local libraries. They also keep abreast of state immunization laws.

Vaccine Policy Institute (VPI)
Kristine M. Severyn, R.Ph., Ph.D., Director
251 West Ridgeway Drive
Dayton, OH 45459
937-435-4750

The Vaccine Policy Institute (formerly Ohio Parents for Vaccine Safety) is a non-profit, educational and research organization devoted to providing parents with information on current government vaccine policies that may affect them and their children. Dr. Severyn, the director, is a registered pharmacist with a Ph.D. in biopharmaceutics. She regularly attends federal vaccine advisory committee meetings in Washington, DC and summarizes these meetings in the VPI newsletter, "Vaccine News". Her information is well researched and accurate. For a minimum $15 donation, you will receive a one-year subscription to the newsletter. Back issues are available for $3.00 each. A complete set of back issue is $30.00 ppd. (12 issues at last count).

Vaccine Research
Josephine Szczesny
P.O. Box 4182
Northbrook, IL 60065-4182
847-564-1403 (4 minute recording)

Josephine Szczesny worked with the late Dr. Robert Mendelsohn. She provides information to health professionals ad parents to help them become aware of the dangers of vaccines. She has compiled "Vaccination Health Hazards: Citations of Articles from Worldwide Medical Journals", $4.00 ppd. (not reviewed) and "Vaccination Dangers" by Josephine Szczesny, $60.00 ppd. (B.1).

Vaccines: Offering Individuals Choice and Education (V.O.I.C.E.)
Lori Morgensen, Founder
P.O. Box 5634
Twin Falls, ID 83303-5634
email: Voice@ltlink.com

VOICE provides vaccine information, especially appropriate for Idaho residents. For a minimum $15.00 donation, you can receive a one-year subscription to the newsletter. Back issues are available for $3.00 each.

Wyoming Vaccine Information Network
Susan Pearce
2184 Hwy 14
Banner, WY 82832
307-737-2325
email: spearce@tctwest.net

They hold monthly meetings on vaccine safety issues and legislative updates.

Defunct Organizations:

The following groups are no longer active. Since some of them are listed as resources in older books, I thought it would be helpful if you know they are now defunct.

Alternatives in Mothering (AIM)
Allenwood, NJ

They are no longer active as of September 1, 1993.

Determined Parents to Stop Hurting Our Tots (DPTSHOT)
Beaverdam, WI

The director, Marge Grant, retired in 1996.

HAVAC
Trabuco Canyon, CA

HAVAC has merged with NVIC and no longer exists as a separate organization effective 1996.

Parents for Freedom of Choice
Plano, TX

This group has been inactive since the summer of 1996. They have reformed under the name Parents Requesting Open Vaccine Education (PROVE), see their listing in this Section.

Natural Immunity Information Network
New York, NY

This group has a new name: New Yorkers for Vaccine Information and Choice. See their listing in this Section.

Ohio Parents for Vaccine Safety
Dayton, OH

This group has a new name: the Vaccine Policy Institute. See their listing in this Section.

South Dakota Raising Immunization Safety Knowledge (SD RISK)
25638 475th Ave.
Renner, SD 57055

They seem to have vanished. (If you know what happened to this group, please let me know.)

Vaccination Alternatives
New York, NY

Ceased operations in December 2001.

2

Health Organizations

American Academy of Pediatrics (AAP)
AAP Publications Dept.
P.O. Box 927
Elk Grove Village, IL 60009-0927
800-433-9016
http://www.aap.org

The AAP issues a free annual catalog of patient educational materials, reference books, and policy statements for its 49,000 pediatric physician members. They publish *The Report of the Committee on Infectious Diseases* (The Red Book), 25th Edition, $89.95 + $10.50 p&h (E) (non-member price). This edition was issued in May 2000. AAP Policy Statements on immunization practices are also available.

American Vegan Society (AVS)
P.O. Box 369
Malaga, NJ 08328
856-694-2887
856-694-2288 Fax

The AVS is a non-profit, educational organization promoting veganism, healthy living, and a compassionate way of life. Membership is $20 per calendar year and includes a subscription to the quarterly magazine "American Vegan". A sample copy is free and includes a current list of all books they sell. They sell many cookbooks, health books, and books on vaccinations, including ones by Harris Coulter, Cynthia Cournoyer, Trevor Gunn, Walene James, Neil Miller, and Randall Neustaedter. The AHIMSA Vaccination issue #36-02 is #3.00 + $1.00 p&h. Free shipping on orders over $5.00.

The Autism Autoimmunity Project
Ray Gallup, President
45 Iroquois Ave.
Lake Hiawatha, NJ 07034
973-299-9162
email: truegrit@gti.net
http://www.gti.net/truegrit

The Autism Autoimmunity Project is a non-profit charity dedicated
to obtaining funding for independent research addressing immune
and immunogenetic abnormalities in autism. They are concerned
about a vaccine cause of autism. They have an informative website
containing research articles on autism. They publish a semi-annual
newsletter. Membership is $25 a year.

Canadian Natural Health Society (CNNS)
P.O. Box 92
Westmount Station
Westmount, Quebec H3Z 2T1
Canada

This health organization promotes the principles and practices of
Natural Hygiene. They publish *Legitimate Immunity Versus Medical
Chaos: Transcending the Futile Dream of Universal Immunization*
by Raymond Obomsawin, $9.95 US + $3.00 US p&h (K).

CDC Vaccine and Autism Web Page
http://www.cdc.gov/nip/vacsafe/concerns/autism

The CDC has set up a new webpage to address parental concerns
about a possible link between vaccines and autism. This page was
set up at the same time as the congressional hearing on autism in
April 2000. The CDC maintains that there is no evidence showing
that vaccines can cause autism.

Center for Empirical Medicine
3324 Palos Verdes Drive North
Palos Verdes Estates, CA 90274
310-378-4597
310-378-7026 Fax
email: emptherapies@earthlink.net
http://www.empiricaltherapies.com

Founded in 1987 by Harris L. Coulter, Ph.D., this publishing and lobbying organization publicizes alternative medical thinking, especially homeopathy. Request a copy of their free book list or visit their website. Among books they publish or sell are: *A Shot in the Dark* by Harris Coulter & Barbara Fisher, $10.95 (B.2); *Vaccination, Social Violence, and Criminality* by Harris Coulter, $14.95 (B.2). Shipping: $3 per book. Dr. Coulter is a medical historian and has written many other health books which may be of interest to you. Check the website for descriptions.

The Couple to Couple League (CCL)
P.O. Box 111184
Cincinnati, OH 45211
513-471-2000
email: ccli@ccli.org
http://www.ccli.org

CCL is a 25-year-old non-profit organization that teaches the Sympto-Thermal Method of Natural Family Planning (NFP) and is dedicated to strengthening marriage and family life. They promote attachment parenting (e.g., the family bed), breastfeeding, and Catholic sexual ethics. Membership is $21 a year and includes their excellent bimonthly newsletter "Family Foundations". Write for their free book catalog.

Families for Early Autism Treatment (FEAT)
http://www.feat.org

FEAT is a non-profit organization providing education, support, and advocacy for the autism community. They have local chapters across the U.S. and Canada. The main website is provided by the northern CA chapter. It has many resources including a search engine on autism. It contains links to other FEAT chapter websites across the U.S. and Canada. They are concerned about a connection between vaccines and autism.

Hepatitis B Foundation
700 East Butler Ave.
Doylestown, PA 18901
215-489-4900
email: info@hepb.org
http://www.hepb.org

This non-profit organization promotes research, treatment, and prevention of chronic hepatitis B. They publish a quarterly newsletter, *B Informed*, that details their activities and provides information on the latest developments in the treatment and prevention of hepatitis B. They strongly support the hepatitis B vaccine and aggressively encourage the establishment of mandatory vaccination laws for hepatitis B. The newsletter keeps track of legislative developments. Every state has a Hepatitis B Program Coordinator, contact them for a list of names, addresses, and phone numbers.

The Holistic Midwifery Institute
Patty Brennan
128 N. Seventh St.
Ann Arbor, MI 48103
734-663-1523
email: patty@holisticmidwifery.org
http://www.holisticmidwifery.org

Patty Brennan is a midwife who gives classes on childbirth preparation, and classes on homeopathy for lactation, children's health, and family health. She also has classes on vaccinations, which covers vaccine safety and effectiveness, prevention and treatment of vaccine reactions, and homeopathic alternatives to vaccines. She will travel to give classes if she has a sponsor. She has a source pack of information titled *Vaccine Choices, Homeopathic Alternatives &*

Parental Rights: A Sourcepack of Information for Healthcare Consumers and Concerned Parents, $22 + $5.00 p&h (A.1).

Homefirst Family Health Forum
Administrative Offices
6400 N Keating
Lincolnwood, IL 60646
800-789-4546 orders
847-679-8336 info
http://www.homefirst.com

Dr. Mayer Eisenstein, MD, JD, MPH has been a doctor for 25 years and is Medical Director of Homefirst Health Services, the largest physician attended home birth service in the U.S. Dr. Eisenstein hosts a weekly nationally syndicated radio talk show called "Family Health Forum". He regularly speaks about vaccinations on his radio show and holds seminars on this topic in the Chicago area.

Homeopathic Educational Services
2124 Kittredge St.
Berkeley, CA 94704
800-359-9051 orders only
510-649-0294 info/catalogs
510-649-1955 fax
email: mail@homeopathic.com
http://www.homeopathic.com

This company specializes in books on homeopathy and related health topics. Their catalog is free. They sell: *The Vaccine Guide* by Randall Neustaedter, $14.95 (A.1); *Vaccination, Social Violence and Criminality* by Harris Coulter, $14.95 (B.2); *A Shot in the Dark* by Harris Coulter & Barbara Fisher, $10.95 (B.2); *A Handbook of Homeopathic Alternatives to Immunisation* by Susan Curtis, $12.00 (I); *Vaccinations? A Review of Risks and Alternatives* by Isaac Golden, $20.00 (I). Shipping: for orders $15.00 or less: $4.50; $15.00 - $29.99: $5.50; $30.00 - $74.99: $6.50.

The Homeopathic College
Dr. Manfred Mueller, DHM, CCH
3622 Lycken Parkway, Suite 3008B
Durham, NC 27707
919-286-0500

Contact them for information on homeopathic immunization and
possible referral to a homeopathic doctor in your area.

International Childbirth Education Association (ICEA)
ICEA Bookcenter
P.O. Box 20048
Minneapolis, MN 55420
800-624-4934 orders only
612-854-8660 catalogs
email: info@icea.org
http://www.icea.org

ICEA, founded in 1960, trains childbirth educators and promotes
family-centered maternity care. They publish ICEA Bookmarks, a
large free catalog containing many books on pregnancy, childbirth,
breastfeeding, parenting, and early childcare, as well as instructional
materials for childbirth educators. Their catalog is also online. They
currently sell: *What Every Parent Should Know About Childhood
Immunization* by Jamie Murphy, $13.95 + $5.00 p&h (A.1).

National Center for Homeopathy
801 North Fairfax St., Suite 306
Alexandria, VA 22314
703-548-7790
703-548-7792 fax
http://www.homeopathic.org

This is a non-profit, educational organization devoted to spreading
homeopathy. Membership is $45 a year and includes a subscription
to "Homeopathy Today" published 11 times a year. An introductory
information packet is $7 and includes a copy of the annual directory
of homeopathic practitioners. They sell: *The Case Against
Immunization* by Richard Moskowitz, $3.00 + $2.00 p&h (B.3).

The National Health Federation
P.O. Box 688
Monrovia, CA 91017
626-357-2181
626-303-0642 fax
http://www.thenhf.com

This 50-year-old organization is dedicated to promoting freedom of choice in health care through education and legislation. Regular membership is $36 a year and includes the magazine "Health Freedom News" published 6 – 10 times a year. They sell an "Immunization Kit" for $25.00 ppd. (B.1). They sell other vaccine and health books. Request a free book list. Their website contains the current "Health Freedom News" and a membership form.

Natural Hygiene, Inc.
Janet Mulford, Director
14-C Mason St.
Rehoboth, MA 02769
508-990-0146
508-979-5811 fax
email: jan@naturalhygieneinc.com
http://www.naturalhygieneinc.com

This is a non-profit educational organization promoting the philosophy of Natural Hygiene. Annual membership is $20 and includes the bimonthly "Journal of Natural Hygiene". Request a copy of their current catalog, which lists all of the health books, videos, and cassettes they sell, including *Vaccines: Are They Really Safe and Effective?* by Neil Miller (A.1); *Vaccination. Social Violence, and Criminality* by Harris Coulter (B.2); and *Immunization: The Reality Behind the Myth* by Walene James (C).

Natural Living Club
Benjamin Russell, Program Director
224 Fulbright Drive
Mountain Home, AR 72653
870-492-5743
email:prof@centurytel.net

This club holds informal meetings in Arkansas on nutrition and
Natural Hygiene. They have reprints of articles available by mail on
the dangers of immunizations. They sell article reprints on Natural
Hygiene and cookbooks. Request their resource list. Mr. Russell
will answers questions via email.

Nature's First Law, Inc.
P.O. Box 900202
San Diego, CA 92190
888-RAW-FOOD toll-free
619-596-7979
email: nature@rawfood.com
http://www.rawfood.com

They sell food and health products based on a raw food and living
foods diet. They also sell health books including ones on vaccinations.

People for Reason in Science and Medicine (PRISM)
Wanda Ballard
P.O. Box 2102
Anaheim, CA 92814
714-995-4889 office
818-342-2396 Sandra Bell, Co-founder

PRISM is a human health advocacy organization opposed to vac-
cines and animal experimentation on scientific grounds. They sell
Vaccination Condemned by Elben (Eleanor McBean) for $5.00 ppd.
(C).

3

Legal Exemptions

The organizations and individuals listed below can provide information for those seeking legal exemptions from vaccinations. Some lawyers are also listed who provide legal help for those seeking exemptions. Many of the organizations listed under Vaccine Organizations can also provide help for those seeking exemptions.

Dorrance Publishing Co., Inc.
Attn: Book Order Dept.
643 Smithfield St.
Pittsburgh, PA 15222
800-788-7654

They publish *Your Personal Guide to Immunization Exemptions*, Grace Girdwain, $10.95 + $2.00 p&h (F).

James R. Filenbaum, Esq.
2 Executive Blvd., Suite 201
Suffern, NY 10901
888-746-8766 toll free
914-357-0020
email: info@immunizationattorney.com
http://www.immunizationattorney.com

Mr. Filenbaum is a lawyer who has been successful in winning court cases allowing parents to obtain legal exemptions for their children; especially religious exemptions based on personal religious beliefs. He practices in New York, Florida, and federal courts. Call for a free consultation to discuss your legal problem and to request a free "immunization packet". He can provide you with legal help on obtaining a religious exemption (for a fee) even if you do not reside in New York. He also handles vaccine injury cases.

Law Office of Stan Lippmann, Ph.D., JD
4500 9th Ave. NE Ste. 300
Seattle, WA 98105
email: Stan@rubella.net
http://www.rubella.net

Mr. Lippmann has a physics degree from John Hopkins University and a law degree from the University of Washington School of Law. He is totally opposed to vaccinations and is active in seeking repeal of mandatory vaccination laws. He has run for public office on an "anti-vaccine" platform. Visit his website to read a law article he wrote arguing for a radical reform of vaccination laws.

Missouri Citizens' Coalition for Freedom in Health Care (MCC-FHC)
P.O. Box 190318
St. Louis, MO 63119-0318
314-968-8755
email: mccfhc@aol.com
http://hometown.aol.com/mccfhc

MCC-FHC is a grassroots organization dedicated to protecting Missouri citizens' rights to freedom in health care through informed and educated choices. The Coalition is currently working to re-instate a philosophical exemption to the Missouri vaccine law for school children, which was legislated away in 1993.

Bonnie Plumeri Franz
815 Knox St.
Ogdensburg, NY 13669
315-393-2950

Ms. Plumeri Franz provides information to New York State residents to help them obtain legal exemptions to vaccinations. She usually refers them to specific court cases or tells them where to look for answers to their particular questions. Send a SASE for her brochure titled "Thirteen Reasons not to Vaccinate".

The Rutherford Institute
Legal Dept.
P.O. Box 7482
Charlottesville, VA 22906-7482
804-978-3888 for information
800-225-1791 orders
email: tristaff@rutherford.org
http://www.rutherford.org

The Rutherford Institute is a legal and educational organization that defends civil liberties and human rights. If your religious exemption request is denied, they may be able to provide legal help.

Special Human Rights Services
Grace Girdwain
8320 S. Nashville Ave.
Burbank, IL 60459-2333

Grace Girdwain has been giving parents advice on how to obtain legal exemptions from vaccination for over 25 years. She will answer questions that you may have on all aspects of obtaining exemptions. Just mail your question to her along with a SASE. She has a brochure available that contains sample exemption forms for $2.00. You can order copies of her book *Your Personal Guide to Immunization Exemptions* for $9.95 + $1.00 p&h (F).

Vaccination Liberation
Walene James, Director
2101 Pallets Ct.
Virginia Beach, VA 23454
757-486-3129
email: vaclib@mindspring.com

This is a grassroots activist organization founded by Walene James, author of *Immunization: The Reality Behind the Myth* (see Greenwood Publications under Publishers) to order, or your local bookstore or health food store. See Section C for the review). The purpose of this group is to work for the repeal of compulsory vaccination laws by educating the public about the problems with these laws, and about theories of alternative health care. Chapter 14 of her book explains methods of contacting people, organizations, and legislators to help realize this goal. For $8.00, you will receive an information packet of vaccine article reprints.

Vaccination Liberation - North Idaho Chapter
Ingri Cassel, President
P.O. Box 1444
Coeur d'Alene, ID 83816
208-255-2307
208-765-8421
email: vaclib@icehouse.net
http://www.vaclib.org

This is the first chapter of Vaccination Liberation to form in the U.S. Basic membership is $20 a year. They publish a quarterly newsletter. Send a SASE for a free info packet.

WashLaw WEB
Washburn University School of Law
1700 College
Topeka, KS 66621
785-231-1185
http://www.washlaw.edu

WashLaw WEB contains links to all fifty states where you can view
State Codes online to find the immunization laws for your state. The
site also contains more than 50 legal directories, provides access to
all known U.S. federal law, a law firm directory, law journals, law
library catalogs, law school links, and other resources.

4

Periodicals

Many of the organizations listed under Vaccines and Health Organizations publish periodicals. The ones contained here are not part of an organization.

Morbidity and Mortality Weekly Report (MMWR)
http://www.cdc.gov/mmwr

The CDC issues all of its current recommendations on vaccines through the MMWR. Subscriptions are $79.00 a year for print copies; however, you can subscribe via email for free at the above website.

Mothering
P.O. Box 1690
Santa Fe, NM 87504-1690
800-984-8116 orders
505-984-8116
505-986-8335 fax
email: info@mothering.com
http://www.mothering.com

"Mothering" calls itself the natural family living magazine. It is published bimonthly. A one-year subscription is $18.95. They regularly feature articles on child health, child rearing, pregnancy, birth, education, and family living. They also routinely publish articles critical of vaccinations. They publish *Vaccination: The Issue of Our Times*, ed. by Peggy O'Mara, $14.95 + $3.00 p&h (not reviewed).

The Vaccine Page: Vaccine News and Database
UniScience News Net, Inc.
1222 SE 46th St., Suite 109
Cape Coral, FL 33904
941-541-3200
http://www.vaccines.com

UniScience runs a website devoted solely to vaccines called The Vaccine Page. It has a search engine to search medical journals for articles on vaccines. It includes: (1) information on adult and pediatric vaccines; (2) information directed to parents, to those traveling, to health practitioners, and to researchers; (3) links to other medical journals and organizations; and (4) the latest news on vaccine research. The Vaccine Page is funded in part by the Bill and Melinda Gates Children's Vaccine Program (see their listing under Vaccine Orgs.).

5

Vaccine Injuries

National Vaccine Injury Compensation Program
Parklawn Building, Room 8A-46
5600 Fishers Lane
Rockville, MD 20857
800-338-2382
301-443-6593
http://bhpr.hrsa.gov/vicp

To file a vaccine injury compensation claim, contact this program. Injuries or deaths resulting from the following vaccines administered after Oct. 1, 1988 are covered under this program: diphtheria, pertussis, tetanus, measles, mumps, rubella, polio (OPV and IPV), and any combination of these. Hib, hepatitis B, and chickenpox were added on August 6, 1997. Deadline for filing claims for injuries or deaths from Hib, hepatitis B, and chickenpox vaccines which occurred from August 6, 1989 to August 5, 1997 was August 6, 1999. Rotavirus vaccine was added to the program on October 22, 1998. The deadline for filing a claim for injuries due to the rotavirus vaccine administered prior to October 22, 1998 was October 22, 2000. On May 22, 2001 pneumococcal conjugate vaccines were added to the program with a retroactive effective date of Dec. 18, 1999. If you think you or your child was damaged by any one of these vaccines you have three years to file a claim. If a death occurred due to a vaccine, you have two years to file a claim.

Call the 800 number (it's a recording) to request an information packet by fax or mail containing instructions on how to file a vaccine injury compensation claim. The packet contains the current Vaccine Injury Table, which lists compensable injuries and the time frame for the appearance of symptoms. If you have further questions after you receive the information packet, they request that you submit them in writing to the above address.

U. S. Court of Federal Claims
717 Madison Place NW
Washington, DC 20005
202-219-9657

If, after you have read the information packet available from the National Vaccine Injury Compensation Program, you want to submit a claim, call or write to the above address and request that the Court Rules and "Guidelines for Practice under the National Vaccine Injury Compensation Program" be sent to you. Claims are submitted to this address.

Vaccine Adverse Event Reporting System (VAERS)
Department of Health and Human Services
P.O. Box 1100
Rockville, MD 20849-1100
800-822-7967
301-217-9660
301-309-6495 Fax
email: info@vaers.org
http://www.vaers.org

The Vaccine Adverse Event Reporting System (VAERS), established in Nov. 1990, is a cooperative program for vaccine safety operated by the CDC and the FDA. If your child has suffered a serious reaction to a vaccine, have your doctor report the reaction on a Vaccine Adverse Event Report form. You can report the reaction yourself by calling VAERS and requesting a report form by mail or fax. They will also answer any questions you may have about filling out the report form. Some adverse reactions require mandatory reporting. Your doctor should have a copy of the Table of Reportable Events Following Immunization, which lists these reactions. If not, you can request one from VAERS.

The new VAERS website wants to serve as a nationwide mechanism by which vaccine adverse events may be reported, analyzed, and made available to the public. They also want to disseminate vaccine safety-related information to parents, healthcare providers, vaccine manufacturers, state vaccine programs, and others.

Attorneys Who Represent Vaccine Injury Cases

It is not mandatory that you have an attorney to place a claim before the NVICP, however, because court rules are very strict, it is highly advised that you retain one. The court reimburses reasonable attorney's fees whether or not you win or lose your case, unless your case is deemed frivolous. I list a few attorneys here, but there are many more across the U.S. with experience in this area. I make no claims as to their abilities.

Conway, Homer & Chin-Caplan, P.C.
16 Shawmut St.
Boston, MA 02116
617-695-1990
email: rhomer@ccandh.com
http://www.ccandh.com

Gage and Moxley
623 W 20th St.
P.O. Box 1223
Cheyenne, WY 82003-1223
307-632-1112
email: VaccineLaw@aol.com
http://www.vaccinelaw.com

They have been active in vaccine injury cases since the start of the NVICP. Their website has information about the NVICP and their current cases.

Altom M. Maglio, P.A.
22 S. Tuttle Ave., Suite 4
Sarasota, FL 34237
941-952-5242
email: assistance@sarasotalaw.com
http://www.sarasotalaw.com

Shoemaker & Horn
9711 Meadowlark Rd.
Vienna, VA 22182
703-281-6395
703-281-5807 Fax
email: shoehorn@bellatlantic.net
http://www.attorneyaccess.net

Located in NVIC'S backyard and close to Washington, DC. Their
website contains helpful information explaining the NVICP.

6

Pediatric Vaccines

Below is a list of each of the universally recommended childhood vaccines indicating their brand name (if any), descriptive titles, ingredients, and manufacturer's names. Manufacturers' addresses follow. Most of these companies also produce other vaccines, but I have not included them here. All information has been obtained from the manufacturer's vaccine package inserts and I note the date of the insert I used.

The pharmaceutical companies who produce vaccines, enclose detailed package inserts with their vaccines. These package inserts, also sometimes referred to as "prescribing information" are important to read, especially for the information they contain regarding contraindications and adverse reactions. They list handling and administering instructions as well as ingredients. A bibliography of studies and references is usually included. There are several ways to obtain these inserts. One of the quickest is to stop at your local public library and look through a copy of the current Physicians Desk Reference (PDR) issued annually. It's big, about three inches thick, and contains detailed product information for hundreds of prescription drugs. Copies of all vaccine package inserts are included in the PDR. You can ask your doctor for inserts from the brands he or she uses. If you have access to the Internet, some vaccine manufacturers let you view the prescribing information online. You can also call the vaccine manufacturers and request these inserts by mail.

A note on Vaccine Ingredients

You'll notice that certain additives are common in most of these vaccines. Thimerosal, a mercury derivative, is sometimes added as a preservative. Because of a report in 1999 showing that the total amount of mercury received by infants by age six months from vaccines exceeded EPA guidelines, manufacturers were asked to develop thimerosal-free hepatitis B vaccines. Formaldehyde is used to inactivate the bacteria in killed, bacterial vaccines. Some residual antibiotics may remain in viral vaccines grown in tissue cultures or cell lines. Aluminum is added to many vaccines to boost the "power" of the vaccine.

Concerning the whole-cell, killed pertussis vaccine, the various manufacturers estimate the amount of "protective units" of pertussis vaccine to be approximately four per 0.5 mL dose. However, as of 1993, the actual number of protective units for the first three doses of DTP, a total of 1.5 mL, could range from 8 to 36 units by law.

Chickenpox (Varicella)

Varivax: varicella virus vaccine live (Oka/Merck). Each 0.5 mL dose contains an minimum of 1350 plaque forming units of Oka/ Merck varicella virus, approximately 25 mg of sucrose, 12.5 mg hydrolyzed gelatin, 3.2 mg sodium chloride, 0.5 mg monosodium L-glutamate, 0.45 mg sodium phosphate dibasic, 0.08 mg potassium phosphate monobasic, 0.08 mg of potassium chloride, residual components of MRC-5 cells including DNA and protein, trace quantities of sodium phosphate monobasic, EDTA, neomycin, and fetal bovine (calf) serum. Contains no preservative. Insert date: 4/99. Manufacturer: Merck.

DT (for children less than 7 years old)

Diphtheria and Tetanus Toxoids Adsorbed, Aluminum Phosphate-adsorbed PUROGENATED. Each 0.5 mL dose contains 12.5 Lf units diphtheria toxoid, 5 Lf units tetanus toxoid, nor more than 0.80 mg aluminum, and a final concentration of thimerosal of 1:10,000. Insert date: 5/88. Manufacturer: Lederle. Distributed by Wyeth-Ayerst.

DTaP (diphtheria, tetanus, and acellular pertussis)

ACEL-IMUNE: Diphtheria and Tetanus Toxoids and Acellular Pertussis Vaccine Adsorbed. Each 0.5 mL dose contains 9 Lf diphtheria toxoid, 5.0 Lf tetanus toxoid, at least 40 µg but not more than 60 µg acellular pertussis vaccine antigens (86% filamentous hemagglutinin (FHA), 8% inactivated pertussis toxin, 4% 69-kilodalton outer membrane protein and 2% type 2 fimbriae), not more than 0.23 mg aluminum hydroxide and aluminum phosphate, not more than 0.02% formaldehyde, final concentration of thimerosal 1:10,000, and possible traces of gelatin and polysorbate 80. Insert date: 1995. Manufacturer: Lederle. Distributed by Wyeth-Ayerst.

Infanrix: Diphtheria and Tetanus Toxoids and Acellular Pertussis Vaccine Adsorbed. Each 0.5 mL dose contains 25 Lf units diphtheria toxoid, 10 Lf units tetanus toxoid, three acellular pertussis antigens (25 mcg pertussis toxin, 25 mcg filamentous hemagglutinin (FHA) and 8 mcg pertactin), not more than 0.625 mg aluminum, 2.5 mg 2-phenoxyethanol as a preservative, 4.5 mg sodium chloride, water for injection, not more than 0.02% formaldehyde, and traces of polysorbate 80 (Tween 80). Insert date: 10/98. Manufacturer: SmithKline Beecham.

Tripedia: Diphtheria and Tetanus Toxoids and Acellular Pertussis Vaccine Adsorbed. Each 0.5 mL dose contains 6.7 Lf of diphtheria toxoid, 5 Lf of tetanus toxoid, 46.8 µg pertussis antigens, not more than 0.17 mg of aluminum, 100 µg (0.02%) residual formaldehyde and thimerosal 1:10,000. Gelatin and polysorbate 80 (Tween-80) were used in production of the pertussis component. Insert date: 9/96. Manufacturer: Aventis Pasteur.

DTP (Diphtheria, tetanus, and whole-cell killed pertussis)

Diphtheria and Tetanus Toxoids and Pertussis Vaccine Adsorbed USP: Each 0.5 mL dose contains 6.7 Lf of diphtheria toxoid, 5 Lf of tetanus toxoid, an estimate of 4 protective units of pertussis vaccine, not more than 0.17 mg of aluminum, not more than 0.02% of residual formaldehyde, and thimerosal concentrated at 1:10,000. Insert date: 4/99. Manufacturer: Connaught Labs. Distributed by Aventis Pasteur.

DTaP and Hib Combined

TriHIBit: ActHIB and DTaP (Tripedia) Combined. This vaccine contains ActHIB, described below under "Hib" and Tripedia described above under "DTaP'. Insert date: 9/96. Manufacturer: Aventis Pasteur.

DTP and Hib Combined

ActHIB with Connaught DPT: This vaccine contains ActHIB, described below under "Hib" and the DPT vaccine manufactured by Connaught Labs, described above under "DPT". Insert date: 9/96. Manufacturer: Connaught and Aventis Pasteur.

Tetramune: Diphtheria and Tetanus Toxoids and Pertussis Vaccine Adsorbed and Haemophilus b Conjugate Vaccine (Diphtheria CRM197 Protein Conjugate). Each 0.5 mL dose contains 12.5 Lf diphtheria toxoid, 5 Lf tetanus toxoid, 10 µg purified Haemophilus b saccharide and approximately 25 µg of CRM197 protein, an esti-mated 4 protective units of pertussis vaccine, not more than 0.85 mg aluminum phosphate, not more than 0.02% residual formaldehyde, and thimerosal 1:10,000. Insert date: 3/93. Manufacturer: Lederle. Distributed by Wyeth-Ayerst.

Hepatitis B

Engerix-B: Hepatitis B Vaccine (recombinant). Each standard 0.5 mL dose contains 10 mcg of hepatitis B surface antigen adsorbed on 0.25 mg aluminum as aluminum hydroxide, not more than 5% yeast (*Saccharomyces cerevisiae*) protein, 4.5 mg sodium chloxide, and phosphate buffers (.44 mg disodium phosphate dihydrate, and 0.35 mg sodium dihydrogen phosphate dihydrate), and thimerosal at 1:20,000. Insert date: 9/99. Manufacturer: SmithKline Beecham.

RECOMBIVAX HB: Hepatitis B Vaccine (recombinant). Each 0.5 mL dose contains 5 mcg of hepatitis B surface antigen adsorbed on 0.25 mg of aluminum as aluminum hydroxide, and not more than 1% yeast (*Saccharomyces cerevisiae*) protein. There are formulations with and without preservative. Those with preservative have thimerosal added at 1:10,000. Insert date: 9/99. Manufacturer: Merck.

Hib (Haemophilus type b)

ActHIB: Haemophilus b Conjugate Vaccine (tetanus toxoid conjugate). Each 0.5 mL dose contains 10 µg of purified capsular polysaccharide (PRP), from Hib strain 1482, conjugated to 24 µg of inactivated tetanus toxoid, and 8.5 % of sucrose. Insert date: 9/96. Manufacturer: Aventis Pasteur.

HibTITER: Haemophilus b Conjugate Vaccine (Diphtheria CRM197 Protein Conjugate). Each 0.5 mL dose contains 10 µg of purified Haemophilus b saccharide and approximately 25 µg of CRM197 protein. Multi-dose vials contain thimerosal 1:10,000. Insert date: 8/93. Manufacturer: Lederle. Distributed by Wyeth-Ayerst.

OmniHIB: Haemophilus b Conjugate Vaccine (Tetanus Toxoid Conjugate). This is the exact same vaccine as ActHIB. It is manufactured by Aventis Pasteur and distributed by SmithKline Beecham.

PedvaxHIB: Haemophilus b Conjugate Vaccine (Meningococcal Protein Conjugate). Each 0.5 mL dose contains 7.5 mcg of Haemophilus b purified capsular polysaccharide (polyribosylribitol phosphate or PRP), 125 mcg of the B11 strain of *Neisseria meningitidis* serogroup B outer membrane protein complex, and 225 mcg of aluminum as aluminum hydroxide, in 0.9% sodium chloride. Now it no longer contains lactose or thimerosal. Insert date: 3/98. Manufacturer: Merck.

ProHIBit: Haemophilus b Conjugate Vaccine (Diphtheria Toxoid Conjugate). Each 0.5 mL dose contains 25 µg of purified capsular polysaccharide (a PRP of the Eagen Hib strain), 18 µg of diphtheria toxoid protein, and thimerosal 1:10,000. Manufacturer: Aventis Pasteur.

Hib and Hepatitis B Combined

COMVAX: Haemophilus b Conjugate (Meningococcal Protein Conjugate) and Hepatitis B (Recombinant) Vaccine. This is a combination of the vaccines, PedvaxHIB, listed under "Hib" above, and RECOMBIVAX HB listed under "Hepatitis B" above. Insert date: 1997. Manufacturer: Merck.

MMR (Measles, Mumps, and Rubella)

M-M-R II: Measles, Mumps, and Rubella Virus Vaccine Live. Each 0.5 mL dose contains not less than 1,000 tissue culture infectious doses (TCID) of measles virus, 20,000 TCID of mumps virus, 1,000 TCID of rubella virus, 14.5 mg sorbitol, sodium phosphate, 1.9 mg sucrose, sodium chloride, 14.5 mg hydrolyzed gelatin, 0.3 mg human albumin, less than 1 ppm fetal bovine serum, other buffer and media ingredients and approximately 25 mcg of neomycin. Contains no preservative. Insert date: 4/99. Manufacturer: Merck. Please note that Merck also makes each of these as separate vaccines.

Pneumococcal

PREVNAR: Pneumococcal 7-valent Conjugate Vaccine (Diphtheria CRM197 Protein). Each 0.5 mL dose contains 2µg of each saccharide for serotypes 4, 9V, 14, 18C, 19F and 23F and 4μg of serotype 6B; app. 20 μg of CRM197 carrier protein; and 0.125 mg of aluminum as aluminum phosphate adjuvant. CRM197 is a nontoxic variant of diphtheria toxin. Manufacturer: Lederle. Distributed by Wyeth-Ayerst.

Polio (killed, IPV)

IPOL: Poliovirus vaccine inactivated, trivalent types 1, 2, 3. Grown in VERO cells (a continuous line of monkey kidney cells) by micro-carrier technique. Each 0.5 mL dose contains 40 D antigen units of type 1 poliovirus (Mahoney), 8 D antigen units of type 2 poliovirus (MEF-1), 32 D antigen units of type 3 poliovirus (Saukett), 0.5% of 2-phenoxyethanol, and a maximum of 0.02% of formaldehyde. Less than 5 ng neomycin, 200 ng streptomycin, and 25 ng polymyxin B per dose may be present. Residual calf serum protein of less than 1 ppm. Insert date: 2/99. Manufacturer: Aventis Pasteur.

Polio (oral, OPV)

ORIMUNE: Poliovirus vaccine live oral trivalent types 1, 3, 3 (Sabin). Each 0.5 mL dose contains a mixture of three types of attenuated polioviruses (types 1, 2, and 3), and less than 25 mcg (micrograms) each of streptomycin and neomycin. It is propagated in monkey kidney cell culture. Insert date: 5/93. Manufacturer: Wyeth-Ayerst.

Rotavirus

RotaShield: Rotavirus vaccine, live, oral, tetravalent. Each vaccine contains four live viruses, a rhesus rotavirus (serotype 3) and three rhesus-human reassortant (DNA mixed together) viruses (serotypes 1, 2, and 4). Each 2.5 mL dose contains equal quantities of each rotavirus serotype. Fetal bovine serum, neomycin sulfate, and amphotericin B are present at a concentration of less that 1 μg per dose. Contains no preservative. Manufacturer: Wyeth-Ayerst. Recalled in October 1999, because of bad adverse effects.

U.S. Vaccine Manufacturers of Pediatric Vaccines

Each time I revise this Guide, it seems another pharmaceutical company has merged with another. Even as I write, new mergers are pending for two of the companies listed below.

Aventis Pasteur
1 Discovery Dr.
Swiftwater, PA 18370-0187
800-822-2463
http://www.us.aventispasteur.com
http:www.vaccineshoppe.com

Vaccines previously manufactured by Connaught Labs and Pasteur Meriux are now being manufactured under the name Aventis Pasteur. Medical professionals can order vaccines online as of April 2000 at their vaccineshoppe.com website. Product information is available on their company website.

Lederle Labs
Division American Cyanamid Corp.
Pearl River, NY 10965

Lederle is now owned by Wyeth-Ayerst Labs and all their vaccines are distributed by them. Contact Wyeth-Ayerst for product information.

Massachusetts Department of Health
Health Biologic Labs
305 South St.
Jamaica Plain, MA 02130
617-983-6400

Two states, Michigan and Massachusetts manufactured their own vaccines. As of 1998, only Massachusetts still does. They manufacture DTP and DT vaccines for use within Massachusetts.

Merck & Co.
Whitehouse Station, NJ
800-672-6372 (product information)
http://www.merck.com
http://www.MerckVaccines.com (for doctors use only)

You can view all their vaccine product inserts on their company website. Patient information about each vaccine and disease is listed, news stories and journal articles, and an online version of the Merck Manual. Health professionals can order vaccines online at the MerckVaccines website.

Glaxo SmithKline Pharmaceuticals
One Franklin Plaza
P.O. Box 7929
Philadelphia, PA 19101-7929
888-825-5249
http://corp.gsk.com
http://www.gskvaccines.com

You can no longer view prescribing information for their vaccines on their website unless you are a health professional.

Wyeth-Ayerst Pharmaceuticals
A Division of American Home Products (AHP)
555 Lancaster Ave.
St. Davids, PA 19087
800-999-9384 (product quality division)
800-934-5556 (product information)
http://www.wyeth.com
http://www.vaccineworld.com

Wyeth-Ayerst Labs distributes vaccines manufactured by Wyeth, Ayerst, and Lederle Labs. View prescribing information online.

7

International Travel

CDC International Travelers' Information Line
877-394-8747
http://www.cdc.gov/travel

By calling the 877 number, you can receive a list of documents
available by fax. Documents available include: (1) vaccine recommendations for children less than two years of age or two years and
older; (2) ordering information for *Health Information for
International Travel,* $22.00 ppd. (J) or call 877-252-1200 to order;
(3) disease risk and prevention information; and (4) current disease
outbreak bulletins. The website lists disease outbreaks by world
regions among other services.

8

Publishers

Alive Books
7436 Fraser Park Dr.
Burnaby, British Columbia V5J 5B9
Canada
800-663-6580

They publish many health books including *Natural Alternatives to Vaccination* by Zoltan Rona, $8.95 US + $4.00 p&h (B.3).

The American Enterprise Institute Press
c/o Publisher Resources, Inc.
1706 Heil Quaker Blvd.
LaVergne, TN 37086
800-937-5557

They published *The Vaccines for Children Program* by Robert Goldberg, $9.95 + $3.50 p&h (G.2).

AUM Publications
Associates in Universal Medicine
Eva Lee Snead, MD
E. Ridgewood Court, Suite 2700
San Antonio, TX 78212
210-826-6613 Fax

AUM publishes *Some Call It "AIDS", I Call It Murder* by Eva Snead, 2 volume set, $29.95 + $4.00 p&h (B.3); *Vaccinations: The Untold Truth* by Y. DeLatte, $14.95 + $1.50 p&h (not reviewed). They also sell audiotapes on vaccination. Ask for a free price list.

Avery Publishing Group
Division of Penguin Putnam
405 Murray Hill Parkway
East Rutherford, NJ 07073
800-788-6262

Avery specializes in health books. They publish *A Shot in the Dark* by Harris Coulter & Barbara L. Fisher, $12.95 + $2.75 p&h (B.2).

Beekman Publishing, Inc.
P.O. Box 888
Woodstock, NY 12498
845-679-2300

They distribute in the U.S. *Vaccination and Immunization: Dangers, Delusions, and Alternatives* by Leon Chaitow, $20.95 + $3.95 p&h (B.3).

The Brookings Institution
Dept. 029
Washington, DC 20042-0029
800-552-5450
http://www.brookings.edu

They distribute books published by Priority Press Publications. You can order *Immunization Dice* by Michael Brody, $10.00 + $4.00 p&h (G.1). They only have a few copies, then the book will be out-of-print.

Earth Healing Products
P.O. Box 11
Dennis, MA 02638
508-385-2055
email: jpmurphy1@neaccess.net

They publish *What Every Parent Should Know About Childhood Immunization* by Jamie Murphy, $15.95 + $2.00 p&h (A.1). Mr.

Murphy has released a song about vaccination titled "The Shot", cassette single, $5.00 + $1.00 p&h. Order both together for $19.95 + $3.25 p&h.

Elsevier Health Science
11830 Westline Industrial Dr.
St. Louis, MO 63146
800-545-2522

They publish *Vaccines* by Stanley Plotkin, 3rd edition, $245.00 hc (E) and *Pocket Guide to Vaccination and Prophylaxis* by Hal Jenson, $23.95 (E). Free shipping if you prepay.

The Grain and Salt Society
Happiness Press
273 Fairway Dr.
Asheville, NC 28805
828-299-9005
800-867-7258
email: topsalt@aol.com
http://www.celtic-seasalt.com

This society promotes the use of sea salt. They also publish various health books. They publish the English edition of *What Price Vaccination?* By Simone Delarue, $15.00 + $3.50 p&h (B.1).

Greenwood Publishing Group, Inc.
88 Post Road West
P.O. Box 5007
Westport, CT 06881-5007
203-226-3571
800-225-5800 orders
http://www.greenwood.com

They publish *Immunization: The Reality Behind the Myth* by Walene James, $26.95 + $6.00 p&h (C) under the imprint Bergin & Garvey.

Hallelujah Acres Publishing
P.O. Box 2388
Shelby, NC 28151
704-481-1700
http://www.hacres.com

They publish *Vaccination: Deception & Tragedy* by Michael Dye,
$8.95 + $5.00 p&h (B.1).

Healthy World Distributing
206 N 4th Ave., Suite 147
Sandpoint, ID 83864
888-508-4787 toll-free orders
http://www.tetrahedron.org

They publish *Emerging Viruses* by Leonard Horowitz, $29.95 hc +
$4.50 p&h (B.3).

IDG Books
1633 Broadway
New York, NY 10019-6785
http://www.idgbooks.com

They publish *Vaccines: What Every Parent Should Know* by Paul
Offit and Louis Bell, ISBN 0-02-863861-1, $12.95 + p&h (A.1).

Integral Aspects, Inc.
110 Eugenie Street West, Suite 439
Windsor, Ontario N8X 4Y6 Canada
519-972-9567
519-942-6861 fax
email: diodati@MNSi.net

They publish *Immunization: History, Ethics, Law, and Health* by
Catherine Diodati $34.98 (C). Shipping: $3.21 for Ontario, $5.50
for the rest of Canada, or $6.80 for U.S. All prices in Canadian

dollars. The book is also available in the U.S. from New Atlantean Press, see Publishers.

Kluwer Academic Publishers

P. O. Box 358
Accord Statión
Hingham, MA 02018-0358
888-640-7378
http://www.wkap.nl

Kluwer bought Plenum Medical Book Co. Plenum published the book *Modern Vaccinology* by Edouard Kurstak, $123.00 + $4.00 p&h if prepaid (D). You can order it from Kluwer.

Koren Publications, Inc.

2026 Chestnut St.
Philadelphia, PA 19103
800-537-3001 orders
215-567-2611
215-567-5601 Fax
http://www.korenpublications.com

Owned by Dr. Tedd Koren, D.C., Koren Publications specializes in patient education products for chiropractors. He offers a selection of books and audio and videotapes on vaccination because of the great interest among chiropractors (and their patients) in this subject. A new report is available titled *Childhood Vaccination: Questions Every Parent Should Ask,* by Dr. Tedd Koren, $13.95, 54 pp,. (not reviewed). Books by Harris Coulter, Jamie Murphy, Walene James, Cynthia Cournoyer, Randall Neustaedter, NVIC, Tim O'Shea, Viera Scheibner, Neil Miller, Robert Mendelsohn, and Grace Girdwain are also available. Request a free copy of "Chiropractic Wellness" his catalog of chiropractic practice building materials, brochures, and related health books or view their catalog online.

Landes Bio Science
810 S. Church St.
Georgetown, TX 78626
512-863-7762
http://www.landesbioscience.com

Landes publishes *Strategies in Vaccine Design* by Gordon Ada, $119.00 + $5.00 p&h (D).

Lisa Lovett, D.C.
Kooyong Road Chiropractic Clinic
86 Kooyong Rd.
Armadale, Victoria 3143
Australia
Phone: 03 509 0233

Immunity: Why Not Keep It? by Lisa Lovett is currently out of print (B.3). However, a second edition is planned.

Marcel Dekker, Inc.
Order Department
185 Cimarron Road
Monticello, NY 12701-5185
800-228-1160
914-796-1772 Fax

They publish *Vaccine Research and Developments: Volume I* by W. C. Koff and H. R. Six, $175.00 hc + $4.00 p&h (D).

The Minimum Price Homeopathic Books
250 "H" St.
P. O. Box 2187
Blaine, WA 98231
800-663-8272 orders
604-597-4757 customer service
604-597-8304 fax
http://www.minimum.com

This company sells homeopathic books primarily to homeopathic and alternative health practitioners. They sell the following immunization books: *A Handbook of Homeopathic Alternatives to Immunisation* by Susan Curtis (I); *Homeopathy and Immunization* by Leslie Speight (I); *Vaccination? A Review of Risks and Alternatives* by Isaac Golden (I); *The Case Against Immunization* by Richard Moskowitz (B.3); *Vaccination and Immunisation* by Leon Chaitow (B.3); *A Shot in the Dark* by Coulter and Fisher (B.2); *Vaccination Social Violence and Criminality* by Harris Coulter (B.2); *Vaccines: Are they Really Safe and Effective?* By Neil Miller (A.1); *Immunization: The Reality behind the Myth* by Walene James ;(C) and *The Vaccine Guide* by Randall Neustaedter (A.1).

National Academy Press
2101 Constitution Ave. NW
Lock Box 285
Washington, DC 20055
888-624-8373
http://www.nap.edu

The National Academy Press publishes all the reports issued by the National Academy of Sciences, National Academy of Engineering, Institute of Medicine, and National Research Council. They publish *Adverse Effects of Pertussis and Rubella Vaccines* by IOM, $44.95 hc (B.2); *Adverse Events Associated with Childhood Vaccines* by IOM, $89.25 (only "printed-on-demand" copies left) (B.1); *The Children's Vaccine Initiative* by IOM, $24.95 (K). Shipping: $4.00 for the first book, $.50 each additional. Their website contains 1000 books online, including these, which you can read free.

New Atlantean Press
P.O. Box 9638
Santa Fe, NM 87504
505-983-1856
800-698-9827 to request a catalog
email: global@new-atlantean.com
http://www.new-atlantean.com
http://thinktwice.com

This press publishes Neil Miller's books: *Vaccines: Are They Really Safe and Effective?* $8.95 (A.1); *Immunization: Theory vs. Reality*, $12.95 (C); and *Immunizations: The People Speak*, $8.95 (B.1). A new book titled, *Vaccine Safety Manual* is available for $10.00 ppd. (not reviewed). They have copies of the immunization laws for each state for $4.00 each and a state-by-state summary of exemption laws, *Vaccine Exemptions*, for $10.00 (F). They also sell many vaccination books from other publishers including books by Coulter, Fisher, Chaitow, James, Neustaedter, Horowitz, Scheibner and Diodati. Call for a free catalog or visit their website. Shipping: 7% or $3.50 minimum.

New West
58 North 13th St.
San Jose, CA 95112
408-298-1800

They publish *The Sanctity of Human Blood* by Tim O'Shea, $6.95 + $1.43 p&h (C).

North Atlantic Books
P.O. Box 12327
Berkeley, CA 94712
800-337-2665
http://www.northatlanticbooks.com

They specialize in health books. A book catalog is $2.00 or free with any order. They publish *The Vaccine Guide* by Randall Neustaedter, $14.95 (A.1) and *Vaccination, Social Violence, and*

Criminality by Harris Coulter, $14.95 (B.2). Shipping: $6.00 first item, $1.50 each additional item.

Oxford University Press, Inc.
Order Department
2001 Evans Road
Cary, NC 27513
800-445-9714 customer service
800-451-7556 orders

They publish all kinds of academic books including *Vaccines and World Health* by Peter Basch, $52.50 hc + $4.25 p&h (K).

Patter Publications
P.O. Box 204
Burlington, IA 52601
319-752-0039
888-513-7770 toll free
208-361-8889 fax
email: patterpublications@yahoo.com
http://www.patterpublications.com

They publish *The Immunization Resource Guide* by Diane Rozario, $13.95 + $2.00 p&h. Quantity discounts available.

Philosophical Publishing House
P. O. Box 220
5916 Clymer Rd.
Quakertown, PA 18951
215-538-5300

Formerly the Humanitarian Publishing Co., they publish various health books. A price list is available free. They publish *The Immune Trio*, $10.00 + $3.50 p&h (B.3).

Publishers Group West
1700 4th St.
Berkeley, CA 54710
800-788-3123
http://www.marlowepub.com

They are the exclusive distributor for books published by Marlowe
& Co. You can order *Take Charge of Your Child's Health* by
George Wootan, $18.95 + p&h (A.2).

Random House, Inc.
Order Department
400 Hahn Rd.
Westminster, MD 21157
800-726-0600 customer service
800-733-3000 orders

They own several other publishing companies, among them Crown
Publishing. You can order *How to Raise a Healthy Child. . . In Spite
of Your Doctor* by Robert Mendelsohn, $6.99 + $4.00 p&h (A.2).

Shoreland Publishing
P.O. Box 13795
Milwaukee, WI 53213-0795
800-433-5256
http://www.shoreland.com

They publish *Travel and Routine Immunizations* by Richard
Thompson, $25.00 + $5.00 p&h for the 2002 edition (J). Published
annually in the spring.

Ian Sinclair
5 Ivy St.
Ryde, NSW 2112
Australia
Phone: 04 296 3900
email: surflover45@hotmail.com
http://www.vaccinationdebate.com

Copies of Ian Sinclair's books *Vaccination: The "Hidden" Facts* are $35.00 AUD ppd. (C) and *Health: The Only Immunity*, $13.00 AUD ppd. (not reviewed).

Dr. Jeffrey Starre, MD
4237 Sunset Blvd.
Steubenville, OH 43952
877-444-7800 toll free

Dr. Starre's book, *Vaccine Free Prevention and Treatment with Homeopathy* (I) is currently out of print. Contact him to see if he will be reprinting it..

SUNY Press
P.O. Box 6525
Ithaca, NY 14851
607-277-2211
800-666-2211 orders
email: info@sunypress.edu
http://www.sunypress.edu

They publish *The Politics of International Health* by William Muraskin, $23.50 hc + $4.00 p&h (K).

Truth Seekers Press
P.O. Box 819
Exmore, VA 23350
757-442-3313

They publish *The Role of Vaccinations in Immune Suppression, Cancer, and AIDS* by Dr. Tedd Spence, $9.00 + $2.25 p&h. (B.3).

Wholistic Practices, Inc.
Heather Muir-Stanley
3617 NW 22nd Terrace
Gainesville, FL 32605
352-375-5553
email: weatbery@mindspring.com

You can purchase Ms. Muir-Stanley's book, *Vaccination and Homeopathic Treatment* for $12.00 ppd. (I).

Acronyms

AAP	American Academy of Pediatrics
ACIP	Advisory Committee on Immunization Practices
CDC	Centers for Disease Control and Prevention
CII	Childhood Immunization Initiative
CVI	Children's Vaccine Initiative
DTP or DPT	diphtheria and tetanus toxoids and whole-cell, killed pertussis vaccine
DTaP	diphtheria and tetanus toxoids and acellular pertussis vaccine
EPI	Expanded Program on Immunization of the WHO
FDA	U.S. Food and Drug Administration
Hib	*Haemophilus influenzae* type b vaccine
IOM	Institute of Medicine
IPV	inactivated polio vaccine
MMR	measles, mumps, and rubella vaccine
NCVIA	National Childhood Vaccine Injury Act of 1986
NIH	National Institutes of Health
NIP	National Immunization Program of the CDC
NVAC	National Vaccine Advisory Committee
NVIC	National Vaccine Information Center
NVICP	National Vaccine Injury Compensation Program
NVP	National Vaccine Plan
NVPO	National Vaccine Program Office
OPV	oral polio vaccine
UNICEF	United Nations Children's Fund
VAERS	Vaccine Adverse Events Reporting System
VCP	Vaccines for Children Program
VIP	Vaccine Information Pamphlet
VIS	Vaccine Information Statement
WHO	World Health Organization

Index

About the Author

Diane Rozario has researched and written about childhood vaccines since 1991, after the birth of her first child. She wrote the first edition of *The Immunization Resource Guide* in 1992. She is a member of the National Vaccine Information Center and the Vaccine Policy Institute.

She has a long-term interest in child health issues. She is Roman Catholic, staunchly pro-life, and a strong supporter of breastfeeding.

Diane and her family live in Iowa where she grew up. She earned a BA in history from Grinnell College in 1985.

She would love to hear your comments about her book. She would especially like to know what you would like to see in future editions. You can contact her via her publisher.

Please visit our website at:

http://www.patterpublications.com
email: patterpublications@yahoo.com

Order Additional copies of

THE IMMUNIZATION RESOURCE GUIDE

For relatives, friends, patients, and members:

Enclose $13.95 + $2.00 p&h. Orders are shipped book rate. (For priority mail, enclose $4.00 for p&h.) Iowa residents, please add appropriate sales tax. US funds only. Satisfaction Guaranteed.

Mail your check or money order to:

Attn: Orders
Patter Publications
P. O. Box 204
Burlington, IA 52601

Or call **800-431-1579** for credit card orders 24 hours a day, 7 days a week.

Call toll free 888-513-7770 to inquire about quantity discounts.

Holy Child Jesus of Good Health: For information about this devotion and to request a holy card, please contact:

Holy Child Jesus of Good Health Devotion
Our Lady of the Holy Spirit Center
5440 Moeller Avenue
Norwood, OH 45212

Order Additional copies of

THE IMMUNIZATION RESOURCE GUIDE

For relatives, friends, patients, and members:

Name: _____

Company: _____

Address: _____

City: _____ State: _____

Zip: _____ Phone: _____

Email: _____

Enclose $13.95 + $2.00 p&h. Orders are shipped book rate. (For priority mail, enclose $4.00 for p&h.) Iowa residents, please add appropriate sales tax. US funds only.

Make your check or money order payable to Patter Publications and mail to:

Attn: Orders
Patter Publications
P. O. Box 204
Burlington, IA 52601

Or call **800-431-1579** for credit card orders 24 hours a day, 7 days a week.

Satisfaction Guaranteed.

Call toll free 888-513-7770 to inquire about quantity discounts.